10

MANUFACTURING TECHNOLOGY RESEARCH



# INTRODUCTION TO INDUSTRIAL TECHNOLOGY

## RESEARCH AND DEVELOPMENT FOR TECHNOLOGICAL PROGRESS

# MANUFACTURING TECHNOLOGY RESEARCH

Additional books in this series can be found on Nova's website under the Series tab.

Additional e-books in this series can be found on Nova's website under the e-book tab.

MANUFACTURING TECHNOLOGY RESEARCH

# INTRODUCTION TO INDUSTRIAL TECHNOLOGY

## RESEARCH AND DEVELOPMENT FOR TECHNOLOGICAL PROGRESS

AKIRA OKADA

NOVINKA

*New York*

For permission to use material from this book please contact us:
Telephone 631-231-7269; Fax 631-231-8175
Web Site: http://www.novapublishers.com



Additional color graphics may be available in the e-book version of this book.

**Library of Congress Cataloging-in-Publication Data**

Okada, Akira, 1960-
Introduction to industrial technology : research and development for technological progress / Akira Okada.
pages cm
Includes bibliographical references and index.
ISBN: 978-1-62081-853-4 (soft cover)
1. Technology. 2. Industries. 3. Technology--Research. 4. Technology--Economic aspects. 5. Technological innovations. 6. Progress. I. Title.
T49.5.O52 2013
338.4'76--dc23

2013003865

*Published by Nova Science Publishers, Inc. † New York*

# CONTENTS

# PREFACE

Industrial technologies have rapidly developed since the Industrial Revolution, and technical progress had been significantly promoted until the 19th century by the great inventors, including James Watt, Alfred Nobel and Thomas Edison. In the 20th century, progress was notably promoted by the activities in the corporate research laboratories, and advanced products, such as nylon and transistors, were developed. Note that technical progress has been closely associated with advances in the relevant scientific area, while the key importance is placed on the generation of ideas, coupled with numerous trial-and-error activities. As a result, large quantities of commodities have been produced at low cost, and the quality of products has been enhanced to achieve a comfortable and convenient living. Market needs are becoming important for promoting further advances since the late 20th century, and sophisticated products to meet the market needs have developed in accordance with the progress in electronic and computer technologies. Most of the sophisticated products, such as portable radio receivers, electronic calculators, portable audio players and personal computers, have developed with the appropriate combinations of existing technologies rather than large-scale investments in the development of novel technology.

Industrial products have progressed with the incremental improvements of conventional products, while the technological advances are associated with progress in science. Successful products have developed with the application of advanced technologies to meet requirements in the market. Understanding human needs and the scientific background around technologies is thus indispensable for further advances in industrial products, and the present publication is intended to overview the essential concepts around industrial technology.

Industrial productions are operated by corporate organizations in most developed countries because competition in the market enhances industrial productivity and improves the quality of products. In Chapter 1, the social and economic issues related to industry are described. Under the market economy, the task of industrial corporations is the provision of products and services to meet market needs, and corporate strategy is critically important for strengthening the company's competitiveness.

Customer needs drive industrial production because the market needs produce the demand for specific industrial products and services. Chapter 2 describes the human needs which produce the demand in the market. As pointed out by Abraham Maslow, human needs form a hierarchy, where the lower layers consist of biological needs that are associated with simple existence, such as water, food and shelter. Our immediate needs are the minimum requirements for human survival, and the immediate task of industries is to provide sufficient amounts of these products. Once the minimum requirements are satisfied, emergent needs are the provision of high-quality products to achieve a comfortable and convenient living. Economic development is important for making daily life more comfortable and convenient, and technological progress improves the quality of industrial products.

Further developments in the economy may achieve the spiritual satisfaction provided by attractive products with sophisticated designs and reliable brand names, and this spiritual satisfaction is enhanced with activities that ensure the individual's future lifestyle and boost prosperity for any descendants. The individual's future life is considerably ensured with the accumulation of wealth and health maintenance in peaceful societies, and the reduction of envisioned risks is preferable for descendants, while a high level of satisfaction is greatly promoted with the self-actuation of activities faithful to their own values. Emergent needs at this stage are associated with technological solutions for assuring the affluent and healthy future life, including medical technology, environmental protection and a sustainable lifestyle. Note that spiritual satisfaction is not the central task of industries but is achieved by good relations with other community members and the self-actuation activities, and economic freedom is of key importance for enhancing the self-actuation activities to conduct a meaningful life faithful to their own values.

Industrial products accepted in the market evolve along with the economic stage, since market needs change with economic development. Improvements in productivity are particularly important for the first stage of economic development to supply sufficient amounts of products, and considerable efforts have been made for achieving process innovation, enabling large-scale production with lower costs. In the second stage of economic development to improve the standard of living and the quality of life, technological development in supplying high-quality products is increasingly important. As a result, advanced products are developed in order to achieve a comfortable lifestyle, and convenient functions are installed in the advanced products. Chapter 3 summarizes the evolution of industrial products, in association with economic development.

Productivity in chemical and biochemical processes has been greatly enhanced with accidental discoveries through trial-and-error approaches. On the other hand, productivity in assembly processes has been improved with the division of labor, and great improvements have been achieved by mechanization and automation. Note that the advanced process of interchangeable parts is a key technology for productivity improvement in the assembly process. Chapter 4 describes the process innovation responsible for the first stage in economic development, in which sufficient amounts of products are supplied.

The deduction of scientific theories promotes technological progress. Maxwell's theory predicts the existence of the electromagnetic wave, and the discovery of nuclear fission in uranium, coupled with the theory of special relativity, predicts the possibility of nuclear weapons. Scientific discoveries during the repetition of trial-and-error approaches towards the development goals directly promote technological advances in the areas of chemical products and industrial materials, represented by the inventions of dynamite, synthetic polymers and transistors. Chapter 5 describes the technological progress leading to the product innovation responsible for the second stage of economic development, in which high-quality products are supplied for comfortable and convenient living.

After achieving a comfortable and convenient lifestyle, spiritual satisfaction, including the assurance of future life, becomes important for industrial products. The accumulation of wealth, while maintaining one's own health, considerably assures one's own future life, and the reduction of envisioned risk is particularly important for any descendants. Once agricultural and industrial products have satisfied the existence needs, the emergent needs are associated with spiritual satisfaction, which includes the maintenance of preferable relations with other community members and the self-actualization activities that may vary depending on the individual's own values. Valuable achievements promoted with enhanced abilities are of key importance for being loved and respected by other group members, and the highest levels of achievements are promoted with the motivation for self-actualization. Chapter 6 describes the technical issues for further advances.

Finally, the present publication is intended to provide essential information for engineers and researchers involved in the research and development of industrial technology, and the relevant issues around industrial technology are summarized. Technical expertise was undoubtedly important for engineers and researchers involved in process innovation and product innovation in the 20th century because the developmental goals were clearly defined, and the priority was placed on promoting the technical abilities. In the next stage of industrial development, additional knowledge around specialized technical issues is increasingly important because a variety of issues are connected with each other, while technical abilities are undoubtedly important. Technological requirements are needed to solve social problems, including the reduction of envisioned risk in this stage, and a variety of issues around industrial technology need to be considered for providing technological solutions. Although the generalized concepts presented here may be a common understanding for experienced industrial engineers engaged in research and development for many years, the consideration of a variety of issues surrounding industrial technology seems to be gaining importance for industrial engineers and scientists in the advanced society of the 21st century.

*Chapter 1*

# INDUSTRY UNDER THE MARKET ECONOMY

Employees engaged in industrial production spend their wages on products and services which maintain their lifestyle, and a self-sufficient economy is becoming rare in modern societies. Accordingly, the workers not only contribute to the product supply, but enhance consumer demand for the products. Mass production generally lowers production costs while the market price is also reduced due to the large amount of products supplied to the market. This is because the transaction price and volume are determined in the equilibrium of supply and demand in the market. Manufacturers are then forced to face severe competition in providing products and services at lower prices, and strategies to enhance the competitiveness of companies are increasingly important under the market economy.

## 1.1. ECONOMY AND SOCIETY

Alvin Toffler described four types of societies; hunting and gathering, settled agricultural, industrial and postindustrial societies, and the transition between them was described with the "waves" concept [1]. The first wave is the Neolithic Revolution, which initiated the transition from hunting and gathering to the settled agricultural society. The Industrial Revolution heralded the second wave, which promoted the transition from the settled agricultural to the industrial society. The third wave that appeared in the middle of the 20th century promoted the transition from the industrial to the postindustrial society. The Neolithic Revolution increased food productivity and the development of food production technology. Due to enhanced productivity, fewer workers were needed in food production, which in turn resulted in an increase in a variety of other products, including clothes, buildings and industrial products. During the Industrial Revolution, industrial production was enhanced by the development of various types of machinery and investments in production facilities have increased the productivity of many industrial products, including fibers and steel.

The Industrial Revolution began in England, where the advanced crop rotation system had increased food production, resulting in population growth, and a large number of wage workers were engaged in the manufacturing sector. An increase in agricultural productivity was associated with technological progress in relevant fields including farming equipment, chemical fertilizers and pesticides. Manufacturing productivity was also enhanced with the division of labor, mechanization and automation. An increase in manufacturing productivity resulted in a decrease in the demand for manual labor, and the transition occurred from industrial to post-industrial society. Walt Rostow described the stages of economic growth from traditional society to the age of mass consumption [2]. In postindustrial societies, the development of valuable products to meet market needs is increasingly important in comparison with production, because production relies on enormous amounts of energy and resources in automated production facilities.

Large quantities of products supplied to the market have satisfied people's minimum requirements and fulfilled their immediate needs. More advanced high-quality products have contributed to the achievement of a comfortable and convenient lifestyle. Technological progress in the products is associated with the accumulation of scientific knowledge coupled with ingenious ideas, and the development of industrial technology has enhanced the quality and quantity of industrial products to satisfy the demand in the market. As a result, most immediate needs are satisfied in the developed countries, where industrial production has facilitated a comfortable and convenient lifestyle. Post-industrial society may thus be defined as an affluent society, in which industrial production satisfies material needs. Daniel Bell has indicated that production is of key importance in industrial societies, and the provision of services is increasingly important in postindustrial societies [3]. Peter Drucker has emphasized the importance of information and knowledge and indicated that organization management is increasingly important because the knowledge worker is inevitably a specialist in a narrow area, and organizations need to manage and maximize the performance of their knowledge workers [4].

Table 1.1 shows the world population, the total general domestic products (GDP), and the GDP per capita until 1998. It is clear that the world economy has developed rapidly since 1820, whereas it had remained relatively static prior to this [5]. Economic growth was greatly promoted with the technological progress that occurred in the areas of transportation and communication [6]. The major transportation systems in 1820 were cargos, barges and sailing ships, and advances in heat engine technology enabled the establishment of a high speed transportation system. Railways and steamboats were realized with the development of steam engines in the 19th century, and the advances in automobiles and aircrafts in the 20th century resulted from the development of internal combustion engines. Handwritten letters were the major communication tools in 1820, and a carrier pigeon was used for rapid communication for a limited distance. Today, simultaneous communication systems, such as telephone, facsimile and electronic mail, are commonly used in a worldwide network, and mass communication systems, such as television broadcasting, are also available.

**Table 1.1. Contours of world development: population, GDP and GDP per capita, in 0 – 1998 [5]**

| | 0 | 1000 | 1820 | 1998 |
|---|---|---|---|---|
| Population (Million) | 230.8 | 268.3 | 1,041.10 | 5,908 |
| GDP (Billion 1990 International Dollars) | 102.5 | 116.8 | 694.3 | 33,726 |
| GDP per capita (1990 International Dollars) | 444 | 435 | 667 | 5,709 |

In addition to transportation and communication infrastructures, productivity has increased with the accumulation of fixed capital and improvements in human capital. Fixed capital, such as machinery, equipment and non-residential structures, has been extensively accumulated since 1820, when mass production was introduced. Primary education became mandatory in advanced countries in the 19th century, and the education period has extended into the 20th century. The global economy has further developed with the progress in the international division of labor and the development of international trade. Advances in transportation technology have reduced the logistics cost, and international investment has encouraged the international division of labor to maximize the production of wealth by focusing on the comparative advantage, as indicated by David Ricardo [7].

In summary, social changes after the Industrial Revolution may be characterized as follows:

(i) Economic growth leads to rapid population growth, and most of the increased numbers of workers are employed in the manufacturing and service sectors.
(ii) Employment in the manufacturing and service sectors requires educated workers, and an increase in productivity has reduced the average working time.
(iii) With economic growth, employment has relatively decreased in agriculture and increased in service industries. Employment in the manufacturing sector has increased in the industrial stage and decreased in the postindustrial stage. This is because industrial development relies on manual labor in the manufacturing sector, whereas technological progress has achieved automated production, operated by limited numbers of employees in postindustrial societies.

## 1.2. Market Economy

Industrial technology originally evolved from making tools to provide the necessities of life, and productivity has been significantly enhanced with the adoption of innovative production processes and advances in mechanization and automation. The number of employees engaged in the production sectors has decreased due to the development of machinery and automation facilities. Automated mass production systems are advantageous in lowering production costs, while requiring large sales volumes to recover the investment.

Demands for consumables, such as fuel and food, remain practically unchanged and predictable because the demands for immediate replenishment are related to the consumption, whereas industrial products which have a long service time have no need for replenishment until they are completely exhausted. Accordingly, the development of advanced products focusing on excellent design and convenience is essential for maintaining the mass production system, as well as facilitating the achievement of a comfortable and convenient lifestyle. The development of attractive products, as well as promotional pricing strategies, enhances customer demand, and the expanding market transaction results in economic growth leading to affluent societies.

### 1.2.1. Supply, Demand and Cost

A variety of products are supplied to the market where currency trading is carried out, and the equilibrium of supply and demand determines the price and trading volume. Figure 1.1 shows the relationship between supply and demand. The greater the demand for the products that are supplied to the market, the higher the transaction price will be. On the contrary, the transaction price will decline when demand is small. Large amounts of products are thus supplied to the market at high transaction prices, while the supplied volume of products with low transaction prices is small. In the competitive market economy, the primary task of industries is to supply valuable products and services at low prices, and the generation of profit is a prerequisite for the continuation of a business operation.

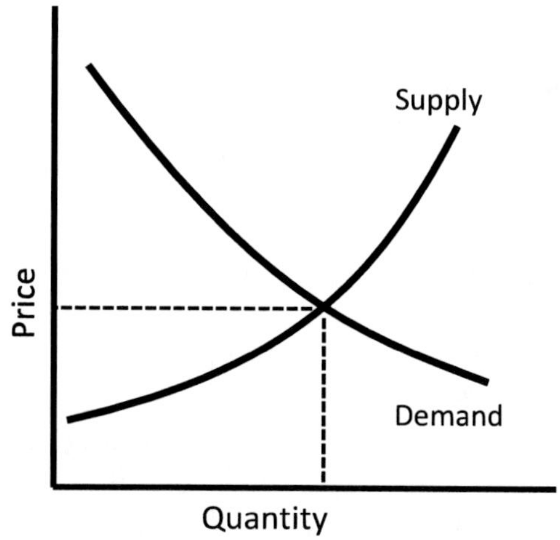


Figure 1.1. Relationship between supply and demand.

Production cost is associated with production volume. Figure 1.2 shows the cost-volume-profit analysis, indicating that the total cost consists of fixed and variable costs. The fixed costs are independent of the production volume, and are associated with support activities and production facilities. The variable costs, such as energy and materials, depend on the production volume. A large production volume reduces the total cost per unit due to the reduction in the fixed cost per unit. Consequently, an increase in the production volume lowers the production cost per unit, while the increased supply to the market may reduce the market price because the market price is determined by the equilibrium of supply and demand.

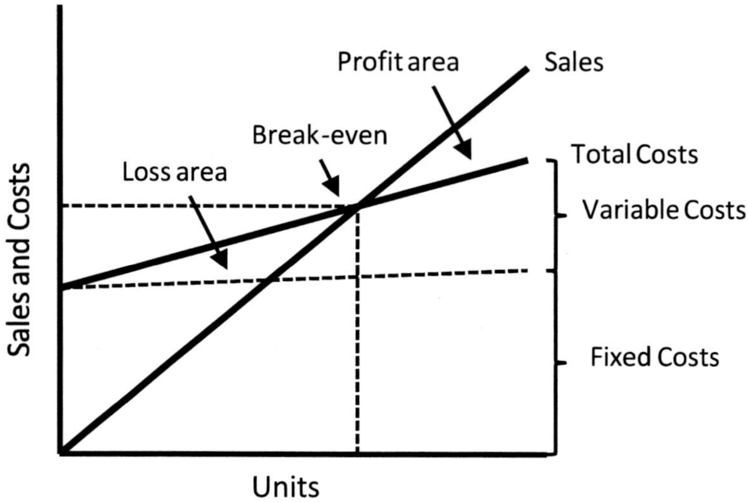


Figure 1.2. Cost-volume-profit analysis.

The decision of whether a new product is to be developed for market launch depends on the relationship between the expected price in the market and the production costs for the expected sales volume. It is noteworthy that the disposal costs of facilities and the compensation costs resulting from unexpected accidents are difficult to include in the analysis because of the uncertainty, and unexpected accidents in chemical plants and nuclear power stations may require additional expenses for the removal of environmental contamination and compensation for injury.

## 1.2.2. Investment and Finance

Increased production requires additional investments in facilities, including manufacturing, logistics and sales. Large-scale facilities promise large profits because the production cost per unit is reduced. Another source of profit comes from the development of exclusive products, and the product differentiation may dominate the market. Therefore, one profitable strategy is to invest in facilities for increasing production at low costs, and another is to promote the developing activities to create valuable products and services.

Investments are usually funded by direct investment through the stock-based business and financial services. An equity investment is recovered with the dividend from the business revenue, and an increase in the corporate value enhances the market capitalization of shares, enabling resale profits from shares.

Funds are normally invested in promising assets to make profits, and the investment makes profits from the increased values of assets. Speculation behaves similarly to the investment, while profits are obtained from changes in the market price. Since the market price under speculation depends on the psychology of speculators, the price is psychologically manipulated. Stock prices can be manipulated with unfounded rumors via newspapers and the Internet. The dominance of the board of directors was an effective strategy for stock price manipulation in the 19th century, when a great profit could be earned with the short selling of shares, combined with the manipulation of information aimed at a decline in stock prices [8]. Good faith is thus an indispensable requirement for reliable organizations, and the behavior of organizations is monitored by citizens and controlled by governmental regulations in democratic societies.

The price of particular shares is intentionally manipulated with large surplus funds, and the purchase of large numbers of shares raises the stock price. Profits are obtained by selling the shares while they maintain high prices, because the manipulated price has no relation to the company's economic activities, and the stock price may return to a reasonable level after the intentional manipulation is terminated. Excessive speculative funds therefore destabilize the market economy, whereas appropriate speculation, such as future contracts to hedge risk, stabilizes the market.

Electronic operation has achieved the international fund transfer instantaneously, and large amounts of surplus funds have been transacted in the international market. The rise in price is intentionally controlled with large amounts of funds injected in particular areas, such as the stock market, currency, bonds, real estate and precious metals, while a sudden crash may occur the moment that funds are withdrawn. Economic boom and the collapse of the bubble economy recur in this way, and the alternate wave of boom and recession in business cycles fluctuates greatly with the flow of speculative funds. The advance in computer technology has facilitated speculative transactions.

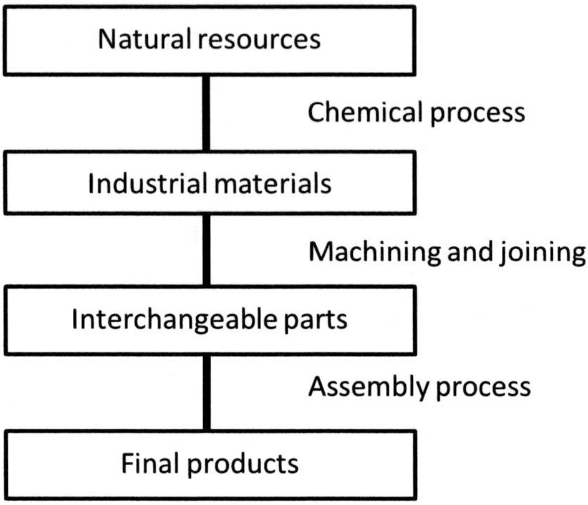


Figure 1.3. Simplified processes in industrial production.

## 1.2.3. Supply Chain and Value Chain

Most industrial products are produced from natural resources through several steps, as simply shown in Figure 1.3. The first step is the extraction process from the natural resources, and the valuable parts are selectively separated from the natural resources to be purified.

Industrial materials produced from purified natural resources are supplied in the form of standardized dimensions, and the chemical compositions and microstructures are adjusted to exhibit excellent material performance. Mechanical parts composing the final product are produced from industrial materials through the forming process, including machining and joining, and interchangeable parts are machined within dimensional tolerances. Final products, manufactured by assembling the parts, are provided for the consumers through wholesalers, distributors and retailers. However, not all of the final products are always manufactured in this way. For example, assembly processes are not used in the production of glass containers and cutlery, and chemical processes are particularly important in the manufacture of some products, including pharmaceuticals, detergents, cosmetics, fertilizers, pesticides, fuels and explosives.

A supply chain is formed by the vertical connection of various stages, typically involving material suppliers, manufacturers, wholesalers, distributors, retailers and customers. A strong connection between the stages benefits in strengthening the supply capability, and vertically integrated companies are at an advantage in steadily providing the final products. The value created in the vertical integration may be divided into individual business units, and strong competitiveness is naturally generated from the strong business unit. Horizontal integration enlarges the particular business unit in order to strengthen the competitiveness because the large business unit is advantageous for cost reduction, and mergers and acquisitions are often undertaken by companies to achieve horizontal integration.

Value creation in business operations may be divided into the contribution of numerous activities, which are comprised of primary and support activities, as described in Porter's value chain [9]. Primary activities are directly related to the value creation, consisting of (i) inbound logistics, (ii) operations, (iii) outbound logistics, (iv) marketing and sales and (v) service, and the support activities comprise (i) procurements, (ii) technology development, (iii) human resource management and (iv) firm infrastructure. The value chain framework is useful for understanding the company's activities leading to its competitive advantage, and the analysis may be used for strategic decisions, such as outsourcing decisions and optimum make-or-buy decisions.

## 1.3. Management and Competitive Strategy

In addition to the endless improvements of products and services, new business creation is indispensable for the survival of companies. Figure 1.4 shows the representative product lifecycle, consisting of introduction, growth, maturity, and decline periods.

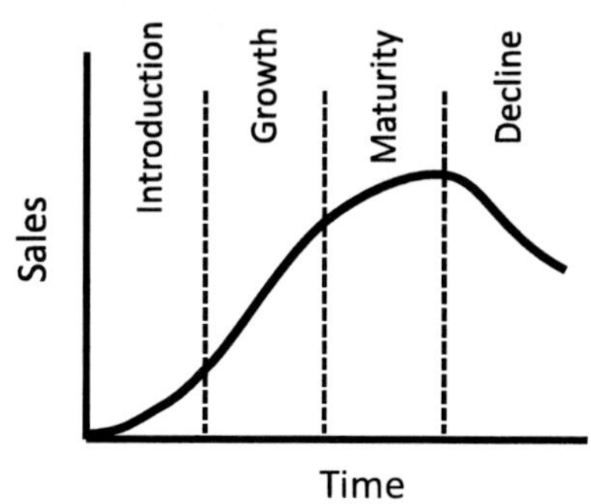


Figure 1.4. Product lifecycle.

The introductory period is characterized by few competitors, high production costs, and a limited number of customers. In the growth period, the products are accepted as meeting specific needs in the market, and the profits are improved.

In the maturity period, the products are well-known in the market while the profit is reduced due to the intensive competition. Both the sales and profits decrease in the subsequent decline period, and the products are regarded as a commodity supplied by low cost manufacturers. Launching new advanced products in the market is thus indispensable for companies continuing production before the end of the product's lifecycle.

### 1.3.1. Marketing

The provision of valuable products and services to meet the customer's needs is an essential activity for business organizations in the market economy, because the organization needs to earn profits for self-sustainment. Marketing is an activity associated with identifying the needs and wants of customers, and innovation is a process used to gain the customer's value [10]. The marketing process normally starts from the situation analysis, which is the identification of opportunities for customer satisfaction. Once the opportunity is identified, a strategic plan is developed, which includes (i) marketing segmentation, (ii) targeting and (iii) positioning. The segmentation is the first step of marketing to divide the market into customer groups, and the purpose of targeting is to choose the customer group to serve. The targeted segment is individually selected for each product and service, and the position of products and services are collated with the customer's needs to find out the benefits for customers. Detailed tactical decisions are comprehensively determined by adjusting controllable parameters, such as product, price, supply chain and promotion.

### 1.3.2. Porter's Five Forces and Competitive Strategy

In a market economy, the existing firms compete with each other to provide valuable products and services at low prices. Fair competition based on good faith for customers and accountability to stakeholders produces social benefits. The government intervenes to ensure social fairness in the market economy, because unfair competition leads to social distortion. Although good faith is unnecessary for society in the market economy, as pointed out by Adam Smith, corporate social responsibility, including the responsibility to society for the effects of organizational activities, is indispensable for valuable organizations in the developed market economy.

Customers receive benefits from a highly competitive market, whereas the industries generally earn low returns due to the severe competition in operative effectiveness. However, not all of the competition is conducted among existing firms providing similar products. New entrants may join the market to supply competitive products and services. Products and services are provided for customer satisfaction, and this satisfaction may be achieved by a less conventional substitute. With the advent of attractive substitutes, customers may switch from the conventional products and services to new substitutes.

Industry earns profits by creating value, and the company's margins are enhanced with operational effectiveness and greatly affected by the prices of purchasing materials from suppliers and selling products to buyers. Accordingly, the competition framework may be described by the five forces proposed by Michael Porter [11]. Porter's five forces are composed of (i) the existing competitive rivalry among existing firms, (ii) the threat of new entrants, (iii) the threat of substitute products or service, (iv) the bargaining power of suppliers, and (v) the bargaining power of buyers.

### 1.3.3. Cost Leadership and Differentiation

According to Michael Porter, the manufacturing industry can choose three competitive strategies for the provision of products; (i) cost leadership to provide products at low prices, (ii) the differentiation of products and (iii) the provision of products focused on a specific segment [11]. Providing products at low prices is a basic requirement for manufacturing companies, and cost leadership is particularly important for competition in commodity products. Production costs include raw materials, energy, labor, and the costs of the depreciation and amortization of fixed assets. The total costs also include logistics and sales. Improvements in manufacturing processes steadily contribute to the reduction of production costs, while the development of innovative processes may drastically reduce production costs.

Business sectors of no profit generation included in indirect sectors are often outsourced after standardizing the business procedures. Resources are usually focused on the business sections of core competence in the value chain, and horizontal integration is promoted with mergers and acquisitions. In addition, low cost operation requires the analysis of the optimal plant location, and the production site is selected to meet the requirements for production including education levels, logistic costs, infrastructures, and political stability. In general, countries with low wage levels are advantageous in supplying commodity products at low costs as long as the minimum requirements for production are satisfied. In contrast, high wage-earning countries may face serious problems of unemployment due to the global optimization in the business locations if the advance is interrupted in the value creation for the sources of differentiation, including innovative technologies and evolutional design.

Differentiation is a strategy for dominating the market by providing valuable products that are supplied by no other companies. Differentiation is promoted with intensive research and development activities. The strategy is usually chosen by companies in an advanced economy, and the profit is obtained by offering exclusive products to differentiate themselves with technology and design. The differentiation strategy is often adopted in research-based companies, and the products usually incorporate advanced technologies. The differentiation is protected with intellectual property rights such as patent, trademark and design, and brand establishment has a strong impact on differentiation. The intensive developmental activities for differentiation certainly lead to an increase in the fixed costs, while new entrants may join the market with limited activities promoted by reverse engineering to analyze the structure and components of the existing products by disassembling.

**The third strategy is to focus the company's resources** on specific segments such as a particular group of customers, products and regions. Note that competitive rivalry is limited in a small segment, and the manufacturers may have a strong bargaining power over the customers. In the case where specific products are exclusively provided, a high market share is expected, while the market volume is small due to the focus on a specific and narrow target. The prompt provision of products and services is in some cases prioritized over low cost, because customers suffering urgent technical problems may demand a prompt solution.

**Table 1.2. The definition of SWOTs**

| | Positive factors | Negative factors |
|---|---|---|
| Internal factors | Strengths | Weaknesses |
| External factors | Opportunities | Threats |

## 1.3.4. Competitive Strategy and SWOT Analysis

Analyzing the competitive situation is important for planning the company's strategy. The activities of companies are affected by external environmental factors, such as political, economic, socio-cultural and technological factors. Some of them work positively as opportunities for companies. However, others work negatively as threats to the company's activities. Factors in the internal environment of companies are divided into strengths and weaknesses, and core competencies significantly contribute to the value creation. Table 1.2 indicates the framework of SWOT analysis, which summarizes the company's Strengths and Weaknesses with Opportunities and Threats in the external environment. In the first step of the analysis, factors affecting the business are classified as being either positive or negative, as well as either internal or external environments, and the situation is summarized in four categories: strengths, weaknesses, opportunities, and threats. Note that the strengths are the origin of the competitive advantage, and a sustainable competitive advantage is supported by the strengths that are difficult to imitate, while strengths due to the rareness of management resources may lead to a temporary competitive advantage.

**Table 1.3. The framework of SWOT analysis**

| | Strengths | Weaknesses |
|---|---|---|
| Opportunities | Strategies to expand the business | Strategies to overcome the weaknesses |
| Threats | Strategies to leverage the strength | Strategies to avoid the worst-case scenario |

The second step is to develop the strategy into four cells produced from four categories as shown in Table 1.3. Competitive strategy has developed to grow the company by capturing the external opportunities, and the company's internal strengths are advantageous in competition. Competitive strategy usually adopts the company's strengths combined with external opportunities. For example, companies with core competency in technological development usually focus on developing advanced products to dominate the market, and production may be outsourced to reduce manufacturing costs. Companies that are competitive in sales may employ a strategy of expanding the sales volume with the company's brand name, with the products being supplied from the contract manufacturers. A company with an advantage in low-cost production may choose a strategy of being a contract manufacturer. In addition to this, the promotion of partnerships between companies is one of the management strategies employed to overcome weaknesses, and business transformation to growth areas leveraging the strengths is one of the business strategies to avoid the threats.

## 1.4. Technological Progress and Innovations

Industrial products have been improved to meet the market needs because products in the market economy are evaluated in terms of benefit and price. Technological progress is basically promoted with the efforts to enhance performance while reducing costs. As shown in Figure 1.5, technological progress typically exhibits S-curve behavior, consisting of the gradual technological progress in the initial stage, the rapid growth in performance in the middle stage, and the gradual growth rate in the final stage.

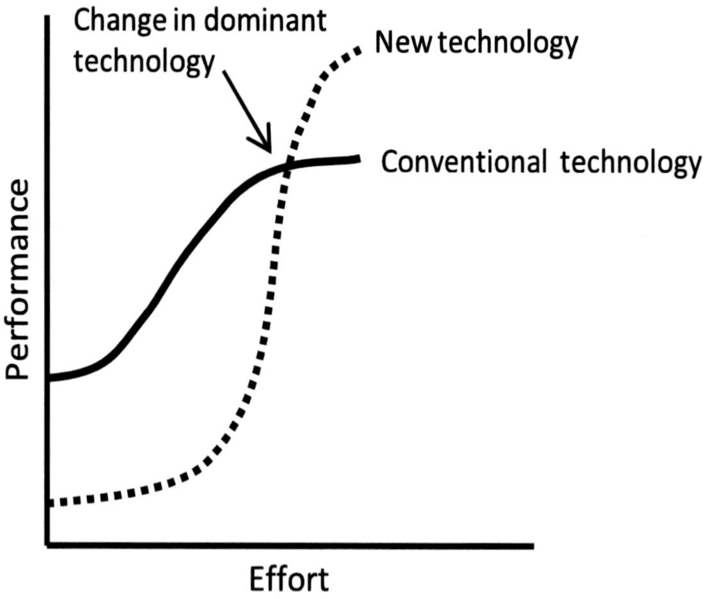


Figure 1.5. Progress in technology exhibiting the S-curve behavior.

As indicated by James Utterback [12], product innovations in the early stage of development are characterized by competition among different methods, and various products are soon converged to the dominant design. Products are then developed within the framework of the dominant design, and innovations dominantly occur in the manufacturing process.

Market needs may be satisfied with substitute products that are based on technology different from the conventional products. As pointed out by Richard Foster [13], the performance of substitute products at the first emergence is very poor in comparison with the conventional technology, because the products are situated in the initial stage of development. The performance of substitutes rapidly increases in the middle stage of development, and the substitute technology may replace the conventional technology. Note that the substitute technology is in many cases not promoted by the established companies, in which the further development of conventional technology is engaged, and the alternation of dominant technology is regarded as the disruptive innovation [14].

## REFERENCES

[1] Toffler, A., *The Third Wave*, Bantam Books, NY, 1980.

[2] Rostow, W. W., *The Stages of Economic Growth: A Non-Communist Manifesto,* Cambridge University Press, Cambridge, 1960.

[3] Bell, D., *The Coming of Post-Industrial Society*, Basic Books, NY, 1973.

[4] Drucker, P. F., *Post-Capitalist Society*, Hyper Collins Publisher, NY, 1993.

[5] Maddison, A., *The World Economy*, OECD Publishing, Paris, 2007.

[6] Maddison, A., *Monitoring the World Economy 1820-1992*, OECD Publishing, Paris, 1995.

[7] Ricardo, D., *On the Principles of Political Economy and Taxation*, John Murray, London, 1817.

[8] Chancellor, E., *Devil Take the Hindmost: A History of Financial Speculation*, Farrar, Straus and Giroux, NY, 1999.

[9] Porter, M. E., *Competitive Advantage: Creating and Sustaining Superior Performance*, Free Press, NY, 1985.

[10] Kotler, P. and Keller, K. L., *Marketing Management 12th Edition*, Prentice Hall, NJ, 2005.

[11] Porter, M. E., *Competitive Strategy: Techniques for Analyzing Industries and Competitors*, Free Press, NY, 1980.

[12] Utterback, J. M., *Mastering the Dynamics of Innovation*, Harvard Business Press, MA, 1994.

[13] Foster, R. N., *Innovation: The Attacker's Advantage*, Summit Books, 1986.

[14] Christensen, C., ***The Innovator's Dilemma***, Harvard Business Press, MA, 1997.

*Chapter 2*

# DEMAND FOR INDUSTRIAL PRODUCTS

Demands are defined as needs alongside purchasing power. No demands are generated in a market economy unless purchasing power accompanies the customers' wants and needs. In a society of large disparity, the demands are largely created by the wealthy, and there exist only very limited demands of the poor. The division of labor enhances the market economy because workers are engaged in the particular parts of production and services in order to purchase the necessities of life. Increased production, accompanied by purchasing power, has enabled the achievement of an affluent life, and material wealth has substantially enhanced individual well-being. In addition, technological progress has improved the quality of products, enabling a comfortable and convenient lifestyle by reducing processing costs.

Further enhancement in well-being requires spiritual satisfaction, and the sophisticated design and brand values are emphasized for the spiritual satisfaction of customers. The need for spiritual satisfaction is related to the extension of human abilities, because spiritual well-being is associated with self-actuation activities to pursue one's own values.

## 2.1. NEEDS AND HAPPINESS

All demands are generated from needs that can be satisfied with the realization of certain requirements, and needs have developed during human evolution. The essential needs, which are common among all living things derived from physiological instinct, are associated with safety and food acquisition. In addition, collective approval, as an intimate member of a group, is indispensable for herd animals, including apes and human beings, since collaborative group work is necessary for the satisfaction of essential needs. Further needs which have developed during human evolution are closely associated with technological developments that have assisted in human survival during the evolution from a chimpanzee's common ancestor. Tools for hunting and defense, such as javelins and sticks, are technical solutions for our human ancestors who discarded the arboreal to start a life on the ground. Clothes, shelter and fire are also technical solutions for essential needs to maintain an adequate body temperature in cold weather, since the fur has been lost during the human evolution.

Numerous trial-and-error activities have been repeatedly performed for developing useful technologies, such as making tools and developing language, and these activities are doubtlessly driven by curiosity. Note that technologies developed during human evolution are not incorporated in human genes as physiological instinct, but are inherited in social culture. Accordingly, advantageous societies are capable of discovering technical solutions for serious problems that have been generated during the evolution of human society, and societies may be characterized with freedom in manifesting curiosity, because the possibility of finding the solution is higher with a greater numbers of attempts.

### 2.1.1. Needs Developed during Human Evolution

All living things have certain essential needs, including the requirement of nutrients and the need to defend themselves against predators. The ability to adapt to a changing environment through biological evolution is an additional requirement for all living things to survive over successive generations as a part of the ecological system. Nutritional intake is mostly conducted with photosynthesis, plant food, and animal food. Chloroplasts in the cells are responsible for photosynthesis, and glucose is synthesized from carbon dioxide and water with photochemical reactions. Chloroplasts have evolved from symbiotic cyanobacteria, and static living things, such as algae and land plants, are the resulting forms of successful symbiosis. Another form of successful symbiosis is phytoplankton, which is a general term for microorganisms performing photosynthesis, breeding on the surface of sea and freshwater to support the bottom of the ecosystem.

Some herbivorous animals choose to ingest large amounts of leaves, such as pandas, and others choose to live with bacteria, involved in a ruminant stomach and a cecum, to degrade cellulose, such as cows and horses. Excellent prey-catching ability is important for carnivores, and the ability consists of detecting, approaching, and catching prey. Developed sensory organs, such as a keen sense of smell, are advantageous for finding prey. An ability for speed is advantageous for approaching prey, and armory, such as sharp claws and fangs, are useful for predation.

On the other hand, defensive strategies against predators may be classified into six categories: (i) to enlarge the body, like elephants and hippopotamuses, (ii) to escape quickly from predators, like herbivorous animals on the prairie, (iii) to hide away, like moles or monkeys, (iv) to protect themselves with tough or prickly skin, like turtles or porcupines, (v) to deter predation with poisonous substances like puffer fish and poisonous mushrooms, and (vi) to fight against predators like bees and scorpions [1]. Defense against predators is generally enhanced with the herd formation due to the early detection of predators and strengthened fighting abilities.

The ancestors of mankind, who biologically separated from the ancestors of chimpanzees around six to seven million years ago to start life on the ground, needed to protect themselves from predators by throwing stones and wielding sticks, while the detailed evolution process leading to modern humans is unclear [2]. The upright bipedal posture seems suitable for stoning and wielding a stick because both feet can be held firmly on the ground, while the behavior of using stones and tree branches as weapons is actually seen in the societies of chimpanzees. As a result, human evolution may be characterized with technological progress inherited through social tradition rather than biological evolution. The cultural characteristics of modern humans are (i) the manufacture and use of tools, (ii) the use of fire, and (iii) the development of language. The biological characteristics are (i) the upright bipedalism, (ii) the loss of fur and (iii) the degeneration of jaws. It is clear that no biological characteristics seem advantageous for human survival, because no other animals having these biological characteristics have achieved successful evolution.

Weapons, originally used for defense against predators to ensure safety, have evolved towards hunting tools, such as spears and lances, and the bow and arrow were also used in battles of war [3]. Discarding fur seems disadvantageous, because fur is useful for protecting skin and the retention of body temperature; however, the possible advantage of losing fur is to cool the body temperature under the blazing sun if sufficient water has been drunk in advance. In order to compensate for the disadvantages caused by the loss of fur, technologies seem to have been developed, including clothes production, shelter construction and heating systems. The evolution of mankind is unusual because the important functions necessary for human survival have been acquired through technological development, including tool production and manipulation, and the technologies are not incorporated in biological genes, but in the society to which it belongs. Therefore, cultural inheritance has played an important role for the survival of the human species, because the acquisition of knowledge and skills during social evolution is not accumulated in the genes, but in social culture [4, 5]. Accordingly, the evolution strategy of humans seems to have shifted from the inheritance of selective genes to cultural inheritance, and the mental structure of feeling happiness through altruistic behavior may have been generated. The development of language is indispensable for acquiring knowledge and skills accumulated in society, while language is thought to have developed for promoting intimate relationships with other group members [6]. The representative cultural inheritances are accumulated in museums, galleries, libraries and computer networks, while the delicate parts of cultural inheritance exist in the language to dominate the mindset.

From the perspective of biological evolution, essential human needs may be summarized as follows. Essential needs consist of food acquisition, defense against predators, and the retention of body temperature, because all living things have to acquire nutrition and defend themselves against predators. The retention of body temperature is an indispensable requirement for cold-blooded animals, such as frogs and insects. Warm-blooded animals in general produce heat, enabling their temperature to remain constant. Human ancestors discarded arboreal lifestyles to start life on the ground, and their valuable fur was lost during evolution. Since then, the serious problems they faced were how to acquire food in the prairie, how to defend themselves from predators, and how to retain their body temperature. The solutions for these problems were provided by technological development. The fabrication and use of tools was effective for hunting and defending, and the body temperature was retained with leather clothes production, shelter construction, and the use of fire.

### 2.1.2. Happiness and Psychological Needs

Abraham Maslow has studied the human motivations of mentally healthy individuals, and has concluded that needs form a hierarchy. Once the lower layer of needs is satisfied, the upper layer of needs takes precedence. Figure

2.1 shows Maslow's hierarchy of needs. Physiological needs, such as air, water, food, clothes and shelter, form the lowest layer of needs to provide the essential requirements for human survival. The second layer is the safety needs, including physical safety and economic safety. The third layer describes the needs consisting of feelings of love and belonging, and this is the need to be accepted as an intimate member in the group. The fourth layer is the esteem needs that are associated with the dominance hierarchy in human society, and is divided into external and internal esteem needs. The external esteem needs represent the lower level that includes social status and recognition, and the internal esteem needs represent the upper level, including self-respect and achievement. According to Maslow, four of the layers of needs are deficiency needs, which are essential for an individual's well-being, and the motivation for the needs diminishes when the needs are satisfied. The top layer is the growth needs for self-actualization to fulfill one's individual potential. The self-actualization needs are rarely satisfied, as Maslow wrote, "Self-actualization rarely happens; certainly in less than 1% of adult population" [7].

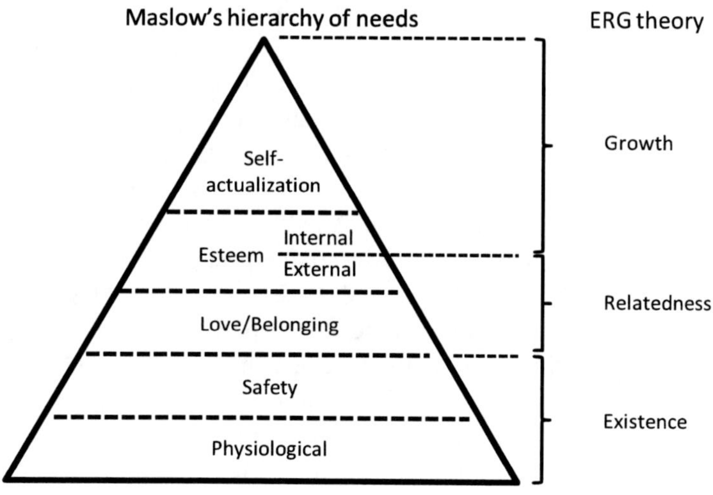


Figure 2.1. Maslow's hierarchy of needs combined with Alderfer's ERG theory [7, 10].

Different types of classification from Maslow's hierarchy of needs have been proposed. Manfred Max-Neef classifies the fundamental human needs into nine categories, including subsistence, protection, affection, understanding, participation, idleness, creation, identity and freedom [8].

Henry Murray divided needs into the primary needs; which are the biological requirements of the body including the need for food, water, air and avoidance of pain, and the secondary needs; such as the need for affection, independence and achievement [9].

Clayton Alderfer proposed the ERG theory, in which Maslow's five layers are simplified into three layers, which are existence, relatedness and growth needs, as shown in Figure 2.1 [10]. The existence needs correspond to Maslow's physiological and safety needs, the relatedness needs correspond to the love and belonging needs and the lower level of esteem needs, and the growth needs correspond to the upper level of esteem needs and the self-actualization needs.

The existence needs are obviously common for all animals, while the existence needs of humans include the retention of body temperature in addition to food acquisition and defense from predators, and tool-making technology has contributed greatly to the existence needs of our human ancestors. The relatedness needs are associated with the collaborative activities of herd animals such as monkeys and apes. Relatedness in the societies of monkeys and apes is strengthened with grooming, whereas relatedness in human societies is strengthened with oral communication using language [6]. The growth needs are common in young humans and animals, and the abilities to prepare for adulthood are extended through play.

John Maynard Keynes classified human needs into absolute needs and relative needs [11]. The absolute needs are satisfied with economic development and the accumulation of wealth, whereas the relative needs to satisfy the desire for superiority are insatiable because the satisfactory levels are determined by the comparison with others. The desire for superiority is associated with the esteem needs, and the display of superiority is common behavior seen in territorial animals. In addition, the need to dominate other group members is seen in the social organization of chickens, Japanese macaques and chimpanzees, and the dominance hierarchy is determined in the group. In animal societies forming a harem, such as walruses, the strongest male dominates the harem, and the strong desire for superiority in human societies may have driven the power struggle over social status and the ethnic domination with force.

Human motivations of mentally healthy individuals have been reported in nursing theory. Florence Nightingale summarized the basic needs of patients [12], and Virginia Henderson chose the fourteen basic needs in daily life activities for nursing [13], which may be classified into nine existence needs, two relatedness needs and three growth needs, as shown in Table 2.1. Note that the basic needs in the nursing theory are consistent with the psychological needs of mentally healthy individuals.

Economic growth enhances levels of happiness. Substantial well-being is growing rapidly with the economic activity at income levels lower than the GDP per capita of US$ 10,000, whereas the level of substantial well-being is rather independent of economic activity above a certain income level [14-16]. The well-being in high-income countries is correlated with the degree of freedom promoted with the social system, in which the personal preference is reflected in the political process, rather than the economic growth [15, 16]. Figure 2.2 schematically shows the well-being dependence on wealth, and the economic growth effectively enhances the well-being in poor countries while the well-being in rich countries is enhanced with the tolerant social system that allows free choice, including social tolerance and political participation.

**Table 2.1. Fourteen basic needs for the fundamentals of nursing [12]**

| | The basic needs of patients | Needs in the ERG theory |
|---|---|---|
| 1 | To breathe normally | Existence needs |
| 2 | To eat and drink adequately | Existence needs |
| 3 | To eliminate bodily wastes | Existence needs |
| 4 | To remove and maintain desirable postures | Existence needs |
| 5 | To sleep and rest | Existence needs |
| 6 | To select suitable clothes; dress and undress | Existence needs |
| 7 | To maintain body temperature within normal range by adjusting clothing and modifying the environment | Existence needs |
| 8 | To keep the body clean and well groomed and protect the integument | Existence needs |
| 9 | To avoid danger in the environment and avoid injuring others | Existence needs |
| 10 | To communicate with others in expressing emotion, needs, fears or opinions | Relatedness needs |
| 11 | To worship according to one's faith | Relatedness needs |
| 12 | To work in such a way that there is a sense of accomplishment | Growth needs |
| 13 | To play or participate in various forms of recreation | Growth needs |
| 14 | To learn, discover, or satisfy the curiosity that leads to normal development and health and use the available health facilities | Growth needs |

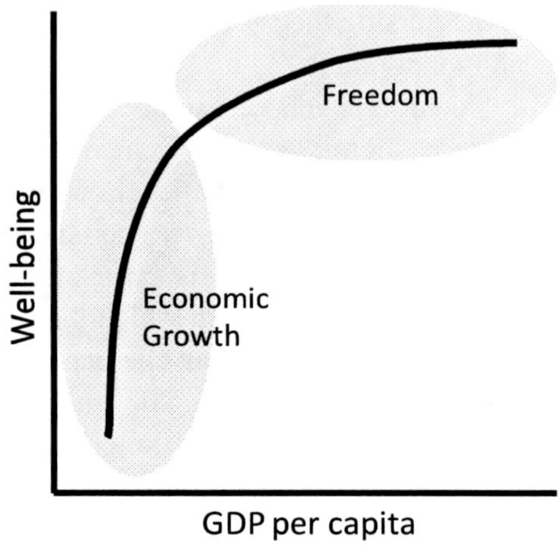


Figure 2.2. Relationship between substantial well-being and GDP per Capita. Economic growth rapidly enhances substantial well-being in the low levels of the economy, and further enhancement of well-being is promoted by freedom in society, rather than the economic growth [14-16].

Daniel Nettle has classified happiness in three levels [17]. Momentary feelings of joy or pleasure are classified as level-one happiness, which produces the transient emotions that arise when listening to music or winning a game. Level-two happiness is subjective well-being, which is enhanced by safety and a healthy life blessed with good friends. Level-two happiness involves judgements about feelings compared to other people and their own pasts. Level-three happiness is achieved by self-actualization activities faithful to one's own values.

Studies of the psychological needs and the classification of happiness imply that economic levels determine three representative life styles. The lowest level of the economy is characterized by a self-sufficient society in which the satisfaction of fundamental deficiency is important; the middle level of the economy is the society of material wealth, in which a comfortable and convenient life is pursued, while people are engaged in playing particular roles to support society. In this stage, economic growth governs the level of substantial well-being. The highest level of the economy is the society of self-actualization, in which people have the freedom to choose what to do and to engage in work which is in keeping with their own values. The society of self-actualization is therefore a tolerant society supported by a democratic social system ensuring the freedom of speech, expression and the press.

## 2.2. Stages of Needs and Economic Development

Foods are supplied by the food industry, clothes are supplied by the textile industry and houses are supplied by the construction industry. Accordingly, the minimum level of physiological needs is immediately fulfilled with a sufficient supply of industrial products. Higher levels of satisfaction are achieved by higher quality products, and advanced industrial products, enabling a comfortable and convenient lifestyle, enhance the level of substantial well-being. Economic development thus creates a society of material wealth to enhance the substantial well-being.

Spiritual aspects are important for further enhancement of substantial well-being. The level-one happiness is promoted with transient emotions and a joyful life, and the feeling of love and belonging satisfies an important part of our deficiency needs. In addition, the advance in the division of labor in modern society forces individuals to engage in a specific part of the social system, and this may cause mental stress. The demands for entertainment and recreation to mitigate the mental stress are thus increasingly important in modern societies of material wealth. In addition, spiritual satisfaction is further enhanced with the activities of reassuring the individual's future life as well as boosting prosperity for his descendants. The highest level of needs is self-actualization driven by the growth motivation to achieve the highest level of happiness promoted with activities faithful to one's own values. Naturally, the activities regarding self-actualization are important for pursuing one's own happiness, and engagement in self-actualization activities is promoted with economic freedom.

Major needs change with the development of the economy, enhanced by technological progress. Immediate needs are important in the lowest level, and technological progress is required for enhancing productivity to supply large amounts of products. In the second level, the quality of products is improved to achieve a comfortable and convenient lifestyle. The spiritual aspects are emphasized in the third level, and products are modified to gratify the mind while the highest level of spiritual satisfaction is achieved with activities associated with self-actualization.

### 2.2.1. Material Wealth

Productivity improvement increases the supply to eliminate the temporary deficiency, and the high-quality products that are produced with technological progress enhance well-being substantially. The additional requirement is to enrich our future life, and the demands are increasing for medical and health care because the individual's future life is considerably ensured with the accumulation of wealth and the maintenance of health in peaceful societies. Another concern is that of leaving valuable contributions to our descendents, and the great interest is directed towards activities associated with the reduction of envisioned risk in the future, including environmental protection, the development of sustainable energy resources and the establishment of sustainable economic systems.

Material wealth has been achieved with enhancing the productivity including technological progress, and the standard of living has been improved to achieve a comfortable and convenient lifestyle. The food supply is enhanced with the development of farming equipment as well as the syntheses of chemical fertilizers and pesticides, and cooking procedures have been facilitated with the progress in kitchenware as well as the development of energy supplies, including the electricity distribution and the gas piping system for fuel. In addition, the development of electric refrigerators has enabled long-term food preservation. Advanced heating systems, including air-conditioners, have provided a comfortable living environment, and the construction of well-insulated houses has improved their heating and cooling efficiencies. The development of synthetic fibers has provided a variety of clothing, and the developments of detergents and electric washing machines facilitate the procedure of cleaning clothes.

The inventions of wheels and ships have strengthened humans' ability to transport, and the invention of characters has enabled the preservation of enormous knowledge as well as communication with written documents. Development in electronic technologies has lead to a new realm of communication, such as telephone, radio and television broadcasting, and advances in audio and video technologies have provided a variety of entertainment, including music and movies.

Once the quality of current life reaches a satisfactory level, major concerns are placed on the health maintenance and the accumulation of wealth to guarantee a future life which sustains an affluent lifestyle. Demands for medical and health care are increasing, particularly in elderly persons, and the preservation of a sustainable environment is a global concern associated with the survival of descendants. One's own life in future is considerably assured by the accumulation of wealth, while a reliable social security system reduces the amount of stockpiling assets required for reassuring the future.

### 2.2.2. Spiritual Satisfaction

Happiness depends on spiritual aspects. Transient emotions are indispensible for a happy life and the feeling of love and belonging is one of the essential needs. Maintaining a good relationship with group members is important for human beings, and the sense of respect given by one's associates raises the level of self-esteem. In addition, a highly stressed lifestyle in modern society requiress rest and refreshment, and the demands for entertainment and recreation are increasing to temporarily refresh the impoverished mind. Entertainment includes a variety of activities in which the audience basically watches the performers and their works in theatres, concerts, exhibitions and television, and the entertainment business sector is steadily growing. Playing sports is a typical recreational activity, and shopping and sightseeing tours also contribute to refreshment. The intake of alcohol and caffeine included in tea and coffee gives a spiritual influence associated with refreshment, while drugs with potent effects are used to enrich the underground economy.

Once the performance of industrial products reaches a satisfactory level, spiritual satisfaction becomes important for the products. Sophisticated design is of key importance for customers in post-industrial societies, while the product design, highly incorporating the artistic aspects, is in general disadvantageous in cost competitiveness because the additional costs are needed for completing the details of products. Brand value is important for reliable companies, and the establishment of high brand value enables companies to maintain a high transaction price under the market economy.

### 2.2.3. Self-Actualization and Growth Motivation

Self-actualization needs are rarely satisfied completely and are rarely exhibited - certainly less than 1% of adult population [7]. However, the activities originated from self-actualization have contributed to the development in human culture, particularly in natural science. Galileo Galilei contributed to the dissemination of scientific thinking supported by quantitative data while his existence needs were threatened by his advocacy for the heliocentric theory. Johannes Kepler was an astrologer and well-known for the laws of planetary motion, while his contribution to astrology was very limited in comparison with his predecessor, Tycho Brahe. The great contribution of an assistant examiner at the Swiss Patent Office, Albert Einstein, was not regarding the evaluation of patent applications but modern physics independent of his responsibilities. These great scientists are obviously promoted by self-actuated growth motivation, not by their job's duties.

Some artists, having established commercial success, tend to pursue self-actualization. Growth-motivated painters such as Katsushika Hokusai and Pablo Picasso proceeded towards the ultimate painting by changing their painting styles. Charles Chaplin produced impressive and didactic movies such as "The Great Dictator" and "Monsieur Verdoux" after his commercial success while he was finally to be expelled from the United States due to such activities. The Beatles concentrated their activities in composing and recording music with innovative sounds without holding concerts after their commercial success.

Some great thoughts are generated from the self-actuated growth motivation. Buddha explored the world of the mind and concluded that liberation from suffering in life is obtained by abandoning desires, and Buddhism is based on his great ideas. John Calvin emphasized faith based on the Bible, and Calvinism justified the way of making a profit through labor and urged the development of capitalism while he was persecuted by the Catholic Church [18]. Some activities promoted with the growth motivation thus led to social progress including natural science, arts and social cultures, and key technologies responsible for enhancing the evolution of human culture, such as the production of stone tools, the use of fire and crop cultivation, may be related to the self-actuation activities.

## REFERENCES

[1] Southwood, R., *The Story of Life*, Oxford University Press, Oxford, 2004.

[2] Crosby, A. W., *Throwing Fire: Projectile Technology through History*, Cambridge University Press, Cambridge, 2002.

[3] Hart, D. and Sussman, R. W., *Man the Hunted: Primates, Predators and Human Evolution*, Westview Press, Colorado, 2005.

[4] Dawkins, R., *The Selfish Gene*, Oxford University Press, Oxford, 1976.

[5] Boyd, R. and Silk, J. B., *How Humans Evolved*, W. W. Norton, NY, 2009.

[6] Dunbar, R., *Grooming, Gossip and the Evolution of Language*, Harvard University Press, MA, 1997.

[7] Maslow, A. H., *Motivation and Personality*, Harper Collins Publishers, NY, 1954.

[8] Max-Neef, M. A., *Human Scale Development*, Apex Press, NY, 1991.

[9] Murray, H. A., *Explorations in Personality*, Oxford University Press, Oxford, 1938.

[10] Alderfer, C. P., *Existence, Relatedness and Growth: Human Needs in Organizational Settings*, Free Press, NY, 1972.

[11] Keynes, J. M., *Economic Possibilities for Our Grandchildren*, Nation and Atheneum, October (1930), reprinted in *Essay in Persuasion*, Macmillan, London, 1931.

[12] Nightingale, F., *Notes on Nursing*, D. Appleton and Company, NY, 1860.

[13] Henderson, V. A., *Basic Principles of Nursing Care*, International Council of Nurses, Geneva, 1960.

[14] Inglehart, R., Foa, R., Peterson, C. and Welzel, C., "Development, Freedom, and Rising Happiness A Global Perspective (1981-2007)," *Perspectives on Psychological Science*, 3 [4] 264-285, 2008.

[15] Veenhoven, R., "Freedom and Happiness a Comparative Study in 46 Nations in the Early 1990's", pp.257-288 in *Culture and Subjective Wellbeing*, Diener, E. and Suh, E. M. ed., MIT Press, Cambridge, MA, 2000.

[16] Frey, B. S. and Stutzer, A., *Happiness and Economics*, Princeton University Press, NJ, 2002.

[17] Nettle, D., *Happiness: The Science behind Your Smile*, Oxford University Press, NY, 2005.

[18] Weber, M., *The Protestant Ethic and the Spirit of Capitalism*, (Translated by Talcott Parsons), Unwin Hyman, London, 1930.

*Chapter 3*

# ADVANCES IN INDUSTRIAL PRODUCTS

Immediate needs that are essential for human existence include water, food, weapons, clothes, shelter and heating, because the essential human activities that are indispensable for survival in a food chain are composed of food acquisition, defense against predators and the retention of body temperature. The primary task of industries is therefore to produce a sufficient amount of industrial products by improving productivity, and the immediate needs are satisfied with the transaction in the market. Once the immediate needs are satisfied, the emergent requirements are to satisfy the existence needs in a way that enhances comfort, convenience and spiritual satisfaction. The secondary task of industries is therefore to develop high-quality products for a comfortable and convenient lifestyle, and the products are incrementally improved. Spiritual satisfaction is not the central task of industries while products of excellent design are advantageous in a competitive market.

Significant advances have been made in the transport and communication technologies, and high-performance equipment for transportation and communications has greatly increased human capabilities. Technological progress in automobiles and aircrafts has contributed to advances in transport technology, and the developments in communication technology, including telephone, television and the Internet, have enhanced the convenience of daily life. Advanced products are designed to meet advanced needs while the product design is to be converged to the dominant design optimized for satisfying needs within the existing technology [1]. Once the technological progress has been made, the provisions of spiritual satisfaction become more important; otherwise, companies often face low-cost competition. Sophisticated product design combined with a reliable brand name spiritually satisfies the existence needs in one's current life, whereas the existence needs in the individual's future life are spiritually satisfied with activities associated with the maintenance of personal health and the accumulation of wealth. In addition, spiritual satisfaction is closely related to activities which satisfy the desire for superiority in the relatedness needs, and the activities which ensure the prosperity of descendants produce the spiritual satisfaction of the current generation. Furthermore, everlasting spiritual satisfaction is achieved by self-actuation activities faithful to one's own values because the self-actuation needs are not deficiency needs but growth needs.

Industrial products have been incrementally advanced to meet the human needs promoted by economic development, and technological innovations have completely changed the conventional products. Table 3.1 lists the representative innovations accompanied with the dominant technology change. Most advances are promoted with the development of electric and electronic technologies to meet the customer's needs, and the innovative technologies have enhanced the functions beneficial for customers. The details in technological progress have been described elsewhere [2-12].

**Table 3.1. Technological innovations accompanied with dominant technology change**

| Conventional technology | Innovative technology | Benefits of innovation |
|---|---|---|
| Phonograph and record player | Magnetic tape recorder | Compact media |
| Gas light | Electric light | Safe and easy operation |
| Ice refrigerator | Electric refrigerator | No need for replenishment of ice |
| Vacuum tube | Transistor | Compact and high durability |
| Mechanical clock | Quartz clock | Compact and accurate |
| Silver halide photography | Digital camera | Onsite image evaluation |
| Typewriter | Personal computer | Elaboration on screen and the incorporation of figures |

## 3.1. Food Products

The immediate requirements for food products are to provide the necessary nutritional components. Starchy food such as grains and potatoes provides the basic calories to the body, and sufficient starchy food enables the meat supply containing high quality proteins because the meat is produced by feeding livestock [13]. Note that the human body requires the intake of nine essential amino acids to synthesize the proteins, and the basic calories are provided by carbohydrates, proteins and fats. In addition, vitamins and minerals are essential for exerting the proper functions, although the deficiency of nutrients as well as the excessive intake could cause health problems and serious diseases. Beriberi is caused by the deficiency of vitamin B1, and the deficiency of vitamin C leads to scurvy. The excessive intake of food leads to the health problems caused by obesity. The risk of heart disease accompanied with hypertension increases with the excess intake of nutrients such as animal fats, salt and sugar. The risk of cancer is greatly increased by the intake of harmful substances such as tobacco. The immediate needs for the food supply are to enhance agricultural production and to develop the preservation technology for food products, and the advanced requirements are to improve the quality of foods.

### 3.1.1. Food Production

In modern societies, most foods are supplied by crop cultivation and the rearing of livestock while some foods are collected by gathering, hunting and fishing. The development of superior varieties is important for enhancing food productivity, and domesticated plants and animals are significantly different from the nature of wild species. The provision of fertilizers enhances crop yields and meat production increases with an increase in feed production for livestock. Therefore, crop cultivation indirectly enhances meat production with the increased feed production.

Varieties of crops and livestock originate from their wild ancestors, and superior varieties have been produced with mutations and mating excellent variations. Radiation breeding increases the possibility of mutation with the production of accidental changes in the DNA. Genetic engineering technically introduces the specific changes in the DNA to produce genetically modified organisms. Progress in genetic engineering techniques has produced new varieties of crops with herbicide tolerance and pest resistance.

Fertilization increases crop yields, and organic fertilizers such as livestock feces and oil cake supply deficient components such as nitrogen, phosphorus and potassium. Chemical fertilizers are chemical compounds soluble in water, and ammonia synthesis from nitrogen in the air has increased the supply of chemical fertilizers. Food productivity has thus been enhanced with the advance in agricultural technology including the development of superior varieties and chemical fertilizers.

### 3.1.2. Food Preservation

Crop preservation starts at harvest time and the meat of slaughtered livestock needs preservation until it is completely consumed. The principle of food preservation is to protect food from decomposition due to attacks from microorganisms such as putrefactive bacteria [14]. The growth of bacteria is suppressed in inadequate environments for bacteria such as low temperatures, low oxygen content, low water content, high osmotic pressure, and acidic solutions. Long-term storage of food is usually carried out in an environment of low temperatures, where bacteria are difficult to grow. The shelf life of food is extended by refrigeration, and frozen food is preserved for a very long period. Cooked food sealed in an airtight container, such as cans and laminated films, prevents bacteria from entering and proliferating inside.

Canned food is most commonly sealed in tin-coated steel, and heat sterilization is normally required prior to the sealing. Vacuum packing is used to preserve food in low atmospheric oxygen pressures, and the shelf life of foods is extended by limiting the growth of bacteria.

**Table 3.2. Methods of food preservation**

| Methods | Major effects |
|---|---|
| Refrigeration | Low temperatures |
| Freezing | Low temperatures |
| Vacuum packing | Low oxygen |
| Drying | Low water contents |
| Smoking | Low water contents |
| Salting | High osmotic pressures |
| Addition of sugar | High osmotic pressures |
| Marinated in vinegar | Acidic solutions |
| Lactic acid fermentation | Acidic solutions |
| Canned food | No bacteria |

Drying, smoking and salting are traditional methods for preserving fish and meat. Cheese, produced by the coagulation of the milk protein casein, is more compact and has a longer shelf life than milk. The shelf life of vegetables is extended by keeping them in marinade because most bacteria are killed in an acid solution. Candied fruit, in which the water is replaced with sugar, prevents the growth of bacteria due to the high osmotic pressure. Fermentation typically converts carbohydrates to alcohols and carbon dioxide, and the process is used to produce alcoholic beverages such as wine and beer. Lactic acid fermentation is applied to the production of yogurt. Table 3.2 summarizes the methods of food preservation. Technological progress in food preservation has stabilized the food supply.

### 3.1.3. High-Quality Foods

In the stage where sufficient food is supplied with the advance in food production and preservation technologies, emergent needs are the delicious and healthy foods for maintaining health. Delicious foods are produced with the breed improvement while the plant's capability of protecting themselves are degraded because the protection strategy of plants is to generate toxic components in the body such as alkaloid, oxalate and cyanide. Advanced crops, in general, need the pesticide to protect them from disease and insect damage.

## 3.2. Clothes

The needs to protect the human skin from cold and mechanical damage resulted from the unfortunate loss of valuable fur. Clothes are used for protecting the skin and retaining the body temperature. Clothes production begins with crop cultivation and livestock breeding since the clothes are produced from fibrous materials such as plant fibers and animal fur, and the development of synthetic fibers has increased the supply of textile products. The textile products are made from the fibrous materials, and the fabrication of high-quality clothes additionally requires the bleaching and dyeing processes. It is important to note that the custom of wearing clean clothes has reduced the infection risk. This has been due to the increased production of clothes and the development of washing technology. The desire for superiority has enhanced the development of high-quality clothes, and self-actualization needs have resulted in the development of uniquely designed clothes.

### 3.2.1. Synthetic Fibers

An increase in food production may result in a decrease in the production of fuels and agriculture-based materials because agricultural products are used for foods, fuels and industrial materials. Since an increase in food production is required for population growth, it is crucial to develop alternative techniques for producing energy resources and industrial materials.

Organic materials have been synthesized from fossil fuels, and new energy resources including fossil fuels and atomic energy have been developed. Biological resources are effectively used for regenerated cellulose fibers, and the synthetic fibers, which are produced from fossil fuels, have developed as substitute products for natural fibers that are provided by plants and animals such as cotton, wool and silk.

Cotton is a typical cellulose-based natural fiber while the available fibrous portions are limited to cotton balls that develop around the seeds. Regenerated cellulose fibers are manufactured from dissolving pulp, and the cupro-ammonium process provides the regenerated cellulose fibers. Cellulose acetate is a class of modified cellulose fibers, consisting of the acetate ester of cellulose developed in 1865. Nylon is the first synthetic fiber of polyamides produced in 1938 as a substitute for silk, and acrylic fibers made of polyacrylonitrile were developed in 1941. Industrial polyester fiber or polyethylene terephthalate (PET) has specific advantages over natural fabrics such as improved wrinkle resistance, durability and high color retention. Technological advances in synthetic polymers have not only resulted in the increased production of clothes but also high-quality plastic products.

### 3.2.2. Spinning, Weaving, Bleaching and Dyeing

Mechanization in the Industrial Revolution greatly enhanced the productivity of the spinning and weaving processes [15]. Advances in the spinning and weaving processes are summarized in Table 3.3. Note that mechanical ingenuity contributed to the first step of the productivity improvement, and the further progress has been made by the employment of huge power sources.

A spinning wheel, which is hand-driven to produce a single thread, is a primitive apparatus for spinning fiber. The advent of multi-spool spinning frames has increased the productivity, and the power sources such as water wheels and steam engines have achieved the large-scale production.

A spinning jenny is a multi-spool spinning frame that was invented by James Hargreaves in 1764, and Richard Arkwright produced a water frame that was a spinning frame powered by a water wheel in 1769. The traditional loom is hand-driven, and hand-weavers could only weave a cloth as wide as their arm span. In 1733, John Kay patented the flying shuttle which allowed a single weaver to produce much wider fabrics, and Edmund Cartwright developed the power loom equipped with a steam engine in 1785.

Bleaching technologies were also advanced in the age of the Industrial Revolution. The traditional bleaching process is comprised of three steps, taking several months for completing the bleaching procedure. The first step is to immerse the cloth in an ash solution, the second is the exposure to sunlight, and the third is the immersion of cloth in a lactic acid produced from milk. The requirement at the time was to shorten the processing time. Dilute sulfuric acid was successfully used in place of lactic acid, and calcium hydroxide was added to the ash solution to shorten the process time for bleaching. The most important progress has been made by the synthesis of bleaching powder, which is a chemically stabilized form of chlorine. The strong bleaching effect of chlorine has been known since its discovery by Carl Wilhelm Scheele in 1774. Chlorine is harmful to the human body and causes damage in the cloth. Investigations on stabilizing the bleaching effect led to the development of bleaching agents instead of sunlight exposure. The bleaching powder, or calcium hypochlorite $Ca\ (ClO)_2$ produced by the chemical reaction between chlorine gas and calcium hydroxide, were patented by Charles Tennant in 1797. The synthesis of chemical substances such as acid, alkali and chlorine compounds for bleaching agent has contributed in this way to shortening the process time for bleaching.

**Table 3.3. Advances in spinning and weaving processes**

| Year | Achievements (Contributor) |
|---|---|
| 1733 | Invention of the flying shuttle to produce wide fabrics (John Kay) |
| 1764 | Invention of multi-spool spinning frame (James Hargreaves) |
| 1769 | Production of spinning frame powered by a water wheel (Richard Arkwright) |
| 1785 | Power loom equipped with a steam engine (Edmund Cartwright) |

In the 19th century, great amounts of coal gas and coke were produced for the gas and steel industry. The dry distillation of coal produces coke, coal gas and coal tar, and the major application of coal tar in the early days was as the preservative for the timber of railroad sleepers. Chemical substances such as aniline and benzene were separated from coal tar, and the application of coal tar was intensively investigated. As a result, William Henry Perkin successfully synthesized a mauve purple aniline dye in 1856, and the synthesized product has replaced the expensive natural dye in the market.

### 3.2.3. Washing Technologies

Healthy living is promoted with adequate sleep and nutrition, and a clean environment reduces the risk of infection. The purification of sewage reduces the risk of infectious diseases in the digestive system such as cholera and dysentery. The removal of fleas and lice is effective for preventing infectious diseases such as plague and borne typhus, and the infection risk is reduced with the custom of keeping the body clean and wearing clean clothes.

Soap is synthesized from caustic soda and fats, and soap production has increased with the development in the manufacturing technology of caustic soda from rock salt. The increased soap production has facilitated laundering to result in the improvement of sanitary conditions. Laundering is the process to separate the dirt from the dirty cloth. The first step is to beat and scrub the cloth in water, and the dirt separated from the dirty cloth is stabilized in water with soap and synthetic detergents. The second step is to rinse the cloth in order to eliminate the dirty water from the cloth. The water is eliminated from the cloth to be dried. Mechanization has facilitated these procedures, and electric washing machines have replaced the human power with electric motors.

## 3.3. Shelters and Housing

The original function of shelters was the protection from cold weather such as cold, rain and wind, and primitive shelters were equipped with a roof, walls and a fireplace for retaining body temperature. The additional function is to strengthen the defensive capability as protection from enemies and criminals. Weapons such as bow and arrows were equipped in the medieval castles, and the nuclear fallout shelters were built in the era of the Cold War. Security guards and the electronic security equipment are becoming important for assuring safety in civilized countries.

Comfortable and convenient functions are installed in upper class shelters, and technological advances have achieved the comfortable living in modern houses equipped with glass windows for day-lighting, electric lighting systems and room temperature control systems within comfortable temperature levels.

Safety and health maintenance for ensuring future life are additional requirements for houses, and the advanced houses have been designed to reduce the risk for fire and earthquakes without using hazard materials. Reinforced concrete structures are advantageous in withstanding earthquakes, and the health risk is reduced with the elimination of hazardous materials, such as asbestos and formaldehyde. Monitoring equipment, including fire alarm and gas leak detectors, are useful for safety assurance, and the fire risk is reduced in the buildings with fire-retardant materials.

Basic requirements for shelters and houses are associated with the existence needs, and the levels of safety and comfort have been raised with economic development. In addition, the construction of conspicuous buildings has been promoted with the desire for superiority.

## 3.4. Energy and Power Sources

Heat generation is indispensible for retaining body temperature and food cooking, and the dry plant has been used for a common heat source. However, the demand is increasing in civilized societies for heat sources because heat is converted to mechanical power with heat engines, and a variety of fossil fuels such as coal, petroleum and natural gas are used for heat engines. The power of heat engines is further converted to electricity with the rotation of electromagnetic generators, and electric power, distributed through the network, is used for lighting, heating and generating mechanical power. The need for energy is to provide sufficient amounts at low costs because enormous energy is required in power generation and transportation, and the major energy sources are fossil fuels and radioactive uranium.

### 3.4.1. Heat Sources

Dry plants are a primitive form of fuel, and livestock feces have been also used for fuel in arid regions. Heat is produced by burning the fuels usually accompaniedby smoke generation. The use of firewood in an enclosed room requires chimney installation for exhausting the smoke, and charcoal, a carbonized form of wood, considerably suppresses the generation of smoke. The needs for residential heating facilities are: (i) to suppress smoke generation, (ii) to reduce the emission of harmful carbon mono-oxide, and (iii) to avert a possible fire risk. Technologies to meet these needs have been developed, including (i) complete combustion without smoke emission by gas heaters and kerosene heaters, (ii) the separation of heating places from heat generation such as central heating, in which the generated heat is distributed to individual rooms, (iii) electric heating generating Joule heat such as electric space heaters and convection heaters and (iv) heat pump systems to warm the building using heat extracted from outdoor air in cold weather.

### 3.4.2. Lamps and Electric Lighting

Burning fuels emit light, and various fuels have been used for lighting. A burning torch is one of the traditional lighting systems that generates a great amount of smoke. Smoke generation depends on the burning conditions and the advance in flame lighting systems. Candles, oil lamps and gas lighting have successfully reduced smoke generation. The most visible light is emitted from high temperature solids, and small carbon particles present in the flame are responsible for light emission. Smoke generation is suppressed with the stabilized combustion of completely consuming the small carbon particles in the flame. In gas lighting, a faint flame is produced because carbon particles are absent due to complete combustion. Installing a gas mantle inside the frame contributes to strong light emissions because solids at high temperatures efficiently emit visible light.

Electric lighting, advantageous because there is no smoke generation, may be classified into three mechanisms [16]. The first mechanism is the light emission from high temperature solids, represented by incandescent light bulbs. The wavelength distribution is close to the black-body radiation. Light emission from discharge tubes is the second mechanism represented by mercury lamps to emit blue-white light and sodium lamps with yellow light, and the quantum states of excited electrons in the vapor materials included in the discharge tube determine the characteristic wavelength of light emission. Visible light emissions from fluorescent lamps are due to the fluorescent materials coated on the inner surface of glass tubes, where ultraviolet light produced by the glow discharge of mercury is converted to visible light.

**Table 3.4. Lighting mechanisms**

| Lighting mechanisms | Example |
|---|---|
| Emission from high temperature solids | Torch, candles, and incandescent light bulbs |
| Discharge tube | Mercury lamps, sodium lamps, and fluorescent lamps |
| P-n junction diodes | LEDs, and OLEDs |

The third mechanism is an emission from the p-n junctions of a diode, and the characteristic wavelength of light is emitted from the coupling of an electron and a positive hole dependent on the quantum levels of semiconductor solids. The p-n junction diodes generate photoemissions resulting from the electronic transition, and the light emitting diodes (LEDs) produce the light, in which the color of light depends on the quantum levels of a semiconductor material. White LEDs produce the mixed light of blue and yellow color, and a part of the blue light emitted from blue LEDs is converted to yellow light with the fluorescent material placed on the tip of a diode. Organic light emitting diodes (OLEDs) are also capable of producing light emissions, and incremental improvements are conducted to enhance the luminous efficacy while reducing the production costs. Table 3.4 lists the major lighting mechanisms.

### 3.4.3. Power Sources and Heat Engines

Various types of power sources are available. Biological power, such as human power and animal power, is produced in the muscle. Water wheels and windmills are traditional power sources, and the rotational motion is mechanically converted to the particular motion required for the mechanism. Heat engines convert heat into mechanical power, and the Carnot cycle theoretically governs the maximum conversion rate.

A steam engine is a reciprocating engine of external combustion. The steam, produced in a boiler, is supplied to the cylinder for pushing up the piston, and the piston is pulled down with the condensation of water vapor. The steam engine is advantageous in fuel diversity while poor in thermal efficiency because a limited part of heat, generated in the boiler, is delivered to the cylinder for reciprocating motion. Internal combustion engines have high thermal efficiency because all the heat, used for mechanical action, is generated inside of a combustion chamber.

Reciprocating internal combustion engines with spark-ignition include gas engines and gasoline engines, and diesel engines are characterized by compression ignition. In diesel engines, the ignition is made by fuel injection into the combustion chamber, where highly compressed air raises the temperature. The high thermal efficiencies of diesel engines are due to high compression ratios, no throttle valves in the inlet system and the combustion under fuel-lean conditions. A steam turbine is an external combustion engine that generates rotary motion from the pressurized steam produced in the boiler. A gas turbine is an internal combustion engine, in which the rotary motion is generated by the high-pressured combustion gas produced in a combustion chamber. Most steam turbines are used for electric power generation, and heat for the boilers is commonly supplied with the combustion of coal or nuclear fission. Gas turbines are used for electric power generation, and jet engines are used for aircrafts. Natural gas is mostly used for the fuel of gas turbines in power plants, whereas liquid fuels are used for aircraft. Representative heat engines are listed in Table 3.5.

**Table 3.5. Heat engines**

| | Internal combustion engines | External combustion engines |
|---|---|---|
| Reciprocating engines | - Gas engines<br>- Gasoline engines<br>- Diesel engines | - Steam engines |
| Turbine engines | - Gas turbine engines | - Steam turbine engines |

A major application for engines is electric power generation and as power sources for transportation system.The appropriate engines are selected for this particular use. Engines for power plants require low cost generation of electric power, and engines for transport machinery are selected in accordance with the characteristics of the transportation systems. As a result, liquid fuels are commonly used for the transportation system including automobiles, ships and airplanes, and most solid and gaseous fuels are used in power stations. In huge power plants, thermal energy for steam turbines is supplied from the combustion of coal or nuclear fission, and natural gas is used for gas turbines. Most of the liquid fuels produced from crude oil are used for a variety of transportation systems, and the crude oil is separated in accordance with the difference in the boiling temperatures. Volatile components are used for gasoline engines in automobiles, and non-volatile components are used for diesel engines in trucks and buses. Jet engines require a specified liquid fuel with sufficient liquidity during flight high in the sky at low temperatures. Fuel oils are used in diesel engines of large vessels, where the fuels are heated in advance to provide the sufficient liquidity for fuel injection.

### 3.4.4. Power Generation and Electric Applicants

Several methods are known for producing electrical energy because the forms of energy are convertible to each other. Piezoelectric elements generate static electricity of high voltage, thermoelectric elements are capable of producing direct current by the temperature gradient, a solar cell is a device of semiconductor diode to produce direct current converted from light energy, and direct current is produced from chemical reactions in batteries and fuel cells. However, most electric power generation is based on the principle of electromagnetic induction. The power is produced in electromechanical generators, in which a magnet rotor is mechanically revolved within the loop of a conducting material and the electric power is generated in the loop [17]. Mechanical power to rotate the generator is often supplied by heat engines such as steam turbines and gas turbines while water wheels and windmills are capable of directly supplying rotational power to generators. Major energy resources are currently fossil fuels. Coal and natural gas are consumed for electric power generation, while petroleum products are mostly consumed by transport machinery. The use of nuclear fuels, despite considerable risk in controlling nuclear reactors, is due to major concerns about the depletion of available fossil fuels.

Electricity has contributed to the realization of a comfortable and convenient life. Electric light bulbs replaced gas lamps in the late 19th century, and communication has advanced with the inventions of the telegraph and telephone. Electric motors produce mechanical power transformed from the electric power supplied from the electrical outlet, and the electric motors have been utilized in convenient appliances such as mechanical fans, vacuum cleaners, electric refrigerators, washing machines and air conditioners [18]. Electric heaters have facilitated food cooking in small appliances such as electric toasters and rice cookers while microwave ovens have utilized the development of the magnetron that emits microwaves to heat the water molecules directly by enhancing molecular vibration. High-performance secondary batteries have promoted the use of portable devices, including digital cameras, mobile phones and laptop computers, and electric displays have contributed to the development of home entertainment devices such as television and video games. Electrical energy is, in particular, advantageous in comparison with the direct mechanical power sources such as horse power and engine power, in which mechanical power is transmitted by the combination of mechanical elements, while electric power is conveniently supplied with an electrical grid connected to power generators.

## 3.5. TRANSPORTATION

Transport technology is not an immediate need necessary for human survival but has greatly contributed to a comfortable and convenient life because it gives humans the ability to transport things. The effort of carrying heavy loads was reduced by using livestock for transportation. Waterborne transportation was enabled by the invention of watercraft such as rafts and boats. Aerial flight was initiated with the invention of hot-air balloons, and the invention of airplane resulted in speedy transportation. In addition, the progress in the transport technologies has enhanced the transactions with distant regions, leading to the global economy. Table 3.6 lists transport technology.

**Table 3.6. Transport technology**

| Transportation | Example |
|---|---|
| Land transport on road | Horse-drawn vehicles and automobiles |
| Land transport on railways | Locomotives and electric trains |
| Waterborne transport | Rafts, boats and ships |
| Air transport | Hot-air balloons, airplanes and helicopters |

### 3.5.1. Railways and Automobiles

The development of land transportation system has expanded the human ability of carrying heavy loads for a long distance. Powerful animals, such as horses, camels and elephants, were successfully used for carrying luggage and passengers on their backs, and the invention of wheels advanced transportation technology, leading to the development of horse-drawn vehicles. The horse-drawn vehicles were mainly used for road services including horse-drawn rail cars while horse-drawn canal boats were used for waterborne transportation. The use of horse is preferable to human power while horses require feed and rest. Land transportation has been advanced with heat engines to replace horses because rest is not necessary for engines as long as fuel is supplied. The invention of steam engines led to transportation by steam boats, steam locomotives and steam automobiles. Further advances in heat engines have resulted in today's land transportation system, including railways and automobiles. Gasoline and diesel engines are the representative power sources while electric motors are commonly used for railroad transportation.

Transport technology has been developed for the rapid transportation system by assuring comfort and safety. Safety assurance is the most important, and two types of safety equipment have been developed. One safety system seeks to prevent serious accidents. The other development is the safety design to reduce the severity of damages in an accident. Passive safety systems such as anti-lock braking systems and electronic stability control have reduced the occurrence of car accidents, and active safety systems such as seatbelts and airbags have mitigated the damage caused by the accident.

### 3.5.2. Watercraft

Advances in watercraft such as ships and boats are associated with the development of power sources. Primitive watercraft such as rafts and boats are driven by human power, sailing ships harness the power of wind, and modern ships are usually driven by screw-propellers, powered by internal combustion engines. The provision of inexpensive means of transportation reduces logistics costs, and the progress in maritime transport technology has reduced transportation costs, resulting in the enhanced global division of labor.

### 3.5.3. Aircraft and Spacecraft

Flying in the sky like a bird became possible with the successful flight of a manned hot-air balloon in 1783. Manned glider flight first took place in 1853, and the success of manned powered flight on an airplane was achieved in 1903. High speed aviation has been advanced with the development of engines. The original power source for airplanes was a gasoline engine to rotate the propellers, which passed the air in a backward direction to propel the body in a forward direction. A jet engine is an advanced power source, and jet propulsion is motion produced by passing a jet of combustion gas in a backward direction to propel the body in the opposite direction of the jet. The flying speed was greatly increased by utilizing jet engines for propelling airplanes while further advances in flying speeds were achieved by the development of rocket engines. Rocket propulsion is similar to jet propulsion with no air intake needed because the motion is produced by the fuel combustion reacting with an oxidizer carried on the craft. Rockets have been used for missiles, launching artificial satellites and manned spacecraft. The first successful manned space flight took place in 1961 and the first manned moon landing was in 1969.

## 3.6. INFORMATION AND COMMUNICATION TECHNOLOGY

Animals surviving in a food chain have the ability to acquire food and to escape from predators. These abilities have been mostly embedded in the physical form of DNA variants as an instinct, whereas the other abilities have to be developed during body growth by learning the skills and knowledge from other group members.

The use of tools has strengthened the physical ability of humans, and communication using language has allowed the sharing of the knowledge and skills acquired from the belonging group. Sensory organs such as eyes and ears provide the primary information, and the information is communicated using language. Accumulated facts are organized in the form of knowledge, and the knowledge that is summarized in the sequence of cause and effect is in particular useful for predicting what happens as a sequence of events.

### 3.6.1. Accumulation of Information and Knowledge

The property of cultural significance is collected in museums, and the valuable information and knowledge are summarized in the form of book to be collected in the libraries. Primitive methods of accumulating information and knowledge were to draw a picture and to memorize the sentences by the storyteller, and the invention of characters has enabled written communication.

Accumulation of visual information was governed by the skills of drawing, painting and sculpture for a long time, and the invention of silver halide photography has resulted in significant progress in visual information technology. Various devices to reproduce the recorded sound have been developed since the invention of the phonograph by Thomas Edison in 1877. Table 3.7 lists the information technology in the area of documents, audio information, and visual information.

**Table 3.7. Information technology**

| Information | Example of the technology |
|---|---|
| Documents | Invention of characters, typewriters and word processors |
| Audio information | Phonographs and magnetic recording |
| Visual information | Silver halide photography, video camera tubes and solid state image sensors |

Advanced information processing has successfully digitalized the visual and audio information as well as text information. Various digital storage devices, including hard discs, CDs, DVDs and flash memory cards, have been developed for storing the digitalized information [19]. Further requirements for information and knowledge are easy access, and the computer network has achieved easy access to the database. The digitalization of data sources is indispensable for computer access, and all the data, including document, audio and visual information, are digitalized to meet the requirement for easy access.

#### *3.6.1.1. Documents*

Technological progress in creating documents is placed on writing speed and elaboration ability. The writing speed is faster in typewriters than hand-writing, and the elaboration ability is greatly advanced with employing the computer technology such as word processers and personal computers using a word processing program. Various keyboard layouts were proposed for the early types of typewriters to avoid the twining of hummers at high typing speeds, and public acceptance has determined the de facto standard for the keyboard layout. Electric typewriters are advantageous in that there is no twining and the high quality of printing due to the same levels of force provided for electric typing. Computer technologies have enabled to modify the document on a display screen before printing, and the word processing software on personal computers has permitted the insertion of visual image data such as figures and photographs into the accumulated documental data.

#### *3.6.1.2. Audio Information*

Microphones produce the electric signals generated in mechanical vibration, and electric speakers convert the electric signals to the sound vibration. The electric signals are stored in the variety of recording devices. In the phonograph recording developed by Thomas Edison, the vibration was directly recorded in the groove carved on the wax cylinder, and the groove was traced with a stylus connected to a vibration plate that generated the sound. Magnetic recording converts the electric signals into the localized magnetization, and the electric current produced from audio signals is sent to the magnetic head having a small gap, where a strong magnetic field is generated at the moment when a large electric current is supplied to the magnetic head. The strong magnetic field produces the local magnetization in the magnetic material provided on the small gap, and the magnetic material for recording is usually supplied in the form of magnetic tapes and magnetic discs. The magnitude of magnetization is detected to reproduce the recorded sound, and the detected signals are amplified for driving speakers.

#### *3.6.1.3. Visual Information*

Glass of a convex shape creates a two-dimensional image on a screen. The imaging technology has advanced with the development of photo-sensitive materials and devices to fix the images. The first generation is the silver halide photography that appeared in the early 19th century. The two-dimensional images produced on the photographic plate are fixed with the photo-chemical reaction so that silver halide is reduced to silver particles exposed under the strong light. As a result, the permanent image is produced from the temporary optical image with the photochemical reduction of silver halide.

Video camera tubes for shooting a television program employ photo-conductive materials, which convert the optical image to the image of electrical conductivity mapping, and the electrical image is converted to the electric signals by scanning the image with an electron beam. With the advances in semiconductor technology, solid state image sensors using miniature diodes were developed for sensing the optical image, and the solid state image sensors are much smaller than the video camera tubes. Along with the development of data storage devices, the solid state image sensors have dominated image recording technology.

The advent of digital cameras replaced the silver halide photography in the 1990s. The digital camera is a camera to record images taken with the imaging device consisting of the solid state image sensors in the form of digital data, and the quality of image has been improved with an increase in the number of pixels of the imaging device, as well as the increased capacity of flash memory for digital data storage. The advantage of digital cameras over traditional silver halide photography is the capability of viewing the image just after taking the photograph.

### 3.6.2. Communication

Ants communicate to each other with numerous different pheromones, and bees communicate by dancing. Humans most commonly communicate with language, and the oral message is transmitted from a speaker to a listener. Communicating with a remote site requires the means to convey the message, and a written message needs to be carried. The written communication has eliminated the requirement for the speaker and listener to be in the same place at the same time, and the message is sent to the receiver in the form of letter. The postal system has developed in conjunction with the transportation system to carry the postal items, and the communication speed is governed by the transportation system. Communication technology has advanced greatly with the evolution of the electrical technology. Information is converted to an electric signal for sending, and the receiver regenerates the original information from the received electric signal.

Electrical messages are sent through wired and wireless transmission systems, and telecommunication has developed with the technological progress in telegraph, telephone and the Internet. The telegraph had the first success in sending text information. The telephone successfully transmitted voice information between remote locations. In addition, the discovery of the electromagnetic wave has led to the broadcasting of radio and television as well as wireless communication using mobile phones. Mass media, including publication and broadcasting, sends information to large segments of the population at the same time. Broadcasting such as radio and television plays a significant part of mass media and also provides audio and video content for entertainment. The progress in entertainment is closely associated with the progress in information technology. Digital information processing has greatly enhanced the convenience of communication, and numerous base stations for mobile phones have been installed to support the packet communication system. This provides a discontinuous communication to share the communication line with many tasks.

### 3.6.3. Entertainment Technologies

In the past, most entertainment was performed in front of an audience. The development of recording and broadcasting technologies has completely changed the form of entertainment. Originally, the audiences had to gather around performers to enjoy a variety of activities. Technological developments have allowed the recording and broadcasting of the performance. Audiences are satisfied with advanced technologies such as movie films and television broadcasting since it is no longer necessary to gather around the performers.

## 3.7. Health and Medical Care

Defense against predators was a serious problem in the early days of human evolution. The development of hunting tools has put mankind on the top of the food chain. An emergent threat was the battle between humans, and numerous people have died in warfare. The threat of war was mitigated by the establishment of international peace, and the disease became the main cause of death. The removal of the cause of infection and the elimination of harmful predators are important for organisms to thrive in the food chain. An emerging issue for individual longevity is the conservation of a healthy environment to eliminate the causes of infection such as pathogens and hazardous chemicals. As a result, the advances in sanitary and medical technologies have contributed to the improvement in the health of the population. Additional requirements are associated with the environmental conservation because all of the existing organisms including humans have evolved to adapt to the environment, and the rapid change in the environment might cause the extinction of existing organisms.

Technical advances in medical care are important for developing vaccines to prevent infection and drug treatments such as antibiotics. Pharmaceuticals are effective for the relief of symptoms, disease prevention and the treatment of the disease. Acetylsalicylic acid and morphine are effective as analgesics, the inoculation of vaccine prevents infection, and antibiotics such as penicillin kill the bacteria that cause infection.

Health monitoring has resulted in early detection and treatment. In addition, the internal structure of the human body can be visualized with the advanced medical inspection equipment such as X-ray computed tomography, ultrasonic imaging, magnetic resonance imaging and positron emission tomography. Health monitoring has reduced the risk of lifestyle diseases because the normal function of biological activities are degraded with the lifestyle diseases. The risk of lifestyle diseases has been considerably reduced with a nutritionally balanced diet, moderate exercise and restrictions on smoking and drinking. There is a great need for advances in medical technology in order to achieve longevity while maintaining personal health in modern societies. Technological progress to promote human evolution may be one of the potential needs for descendents.

## REFERENCES

[1] Utterback, J. M., *Mastering the Dynamics of Innovation*, Harvard Business Press, MA, 1994.

[2] Forbes, R. J., *Studies in Ancient Technology,* Brill Academic Pub., MA, 1955-1964.

[3] Singer, C. J., *A History of Technology*, Clarendon Press, Oxford, 1954-1984.

[4] Forbes, R. J., *Man, the Maker: A History of Technology and Engineering*, Abelard-Schuman, London, 1958.

[5] Derry, T. K. and Williams, T. I., *A Short History of Technology: From the Earliest Times to A. D. 1900*, Oxford University Press, Oxford, 1960.

[6] Armytage, W. H. G., *A Social History of Engineering*, Faber and Faber, London, 1961.

[7] Forbes, R. J. and Dijksterhuis, E. J., *A History of Science and Technology*, Penguin Books, London, 1963.

[8] Lilley, S., *Men, Machines and History*, Lawrence and Wishart, London, 1965.

[9] Burke, J., *Connections,* Macmillan, London, 1978.

[10] Pacey, A., *Technology in World Civilization*, MIT Press, MA, 1990.

[11] Landes, D. S., *The Unbound Prometheus: Technological Change and Industrial Development in Western Europe from 1750 to the Present*, Cambridge University Press, Cambridge, 1969.

[12] Williams, T. I., *A Short History of Twentieth-Century Technology,* Oxford University Press, Oxford, 1982.

[13] Heiser Jr., C. B., *Seed to Civilization*, Indo American Books, Delhi, 2007.

[14] Potter, N. N., *Food Science*, Springer, Berlin, 1999.

[15] Chapman, S. D., *The Cotton Industry in the Industrial Revolution*, Macmillan, London, 1972.

[16] Žukauskas, A. and Shur, M. S., *Introduction to Solid-State Lighting*, Wiley-Interscience, NY, 2002.
[17] Hughes, T. P., *Networks of Power: Electrification in Western Society, 1880-1930*, Johns Hopkins Press, Baltimore, 1983.
[18] Hughes, A. and MacLoud, D., *Electric Motors and Drives: Fundamentals, Types and Applications,* Newnes, Oxford, 2005.
[19] Piramanayagam, S. N. and Chong, T. C., *Developments in Data Storage: Materials Perspective*, Wiley-IEEE Press, NJ, 2011.

*Chapter 4*

# PROCESS INNOVATION

The primary task of industries is to satisfy immediate needs by supplying sufficient necessities for life. The production of agriculture, metallurgy and chemical products have increased with the development of innovative processes. Agricultural production has increased with a variety of technological advances, including irrigation farming, crop rotation system and advanced machineries for cultivation, and selective breeding has produced excellent crops and livestock. This has improved the quality of foods along with the development of fertilizer and pesticide. Metallurgical productivity has increased with the development of furnaces to generate high temperatures as well as technological progress in the separation and purification processes. In addition, the productivity in steelmaking has increased with the technological advances in furnaces such as the blast furnace and the Bessemer converter. Chemical production has advanced with the discoveries of innovative processes, and the process evolution in basic chemicals such as sulfuric acid, caustic soda and ammonia has resulted in more sophisticated ones that reduce the environmental impacts with less dependence on the scarcity of resources.

Further increases in production require the technological development in the utilization of abundant resources because productivity improvements may result in the depletion of available resources. Iron production in the age of the Industrial Revolution was limited by charcoal production, and the iron production was further enhanced with an advanced process using coke as an alternative to charcoal. Possible depletion of natural minerals used for nitrogen fertilizer was a serious problem at the end of the 19th century, and the solution was provided by the development of chemical fertilizers to improve atmospheric nitrogen. Technological development employing abundant natural resources has thus enhanced industrial production.

Interchangeable parts are combined together to produce the final products in the modern assembly processes, and the productivity has increased with the rationalization in assembly and parts manufacturing. Low cost production per unit is achieved with the investment in large-scale production facilities equipped with automated manufacturing machineries if the investment is recovered by mass marketing.

## 4.1. Promoting Variety in Available Resources

Natural resources are directly consumed for food, fuel and making useful things including tools, clothes and shelter. Food is collected from the edible parts of organic resources, and the edible portion increases by cooking with fire. Hunger risk is reduced with the food supply that is stabilized by the development of food preservation technology. Burnable parts in natural resources are capable of directly supplying fuels while some of the burnable parts are further modified with drying and cutting for the provision of firewood as well as the carbonization for charcoal production. Before industrial development, the necessities of life had been directly produced from natural resources and gathered from the useful parts in plants, animals and stones. Even today, some important industrial products such as timber, cotton fiber and leather are directly produced from useful plants and animals, whereas most industrial products such as steel, cement and glass are chemically synthesized from mineral resources. Figure 4.1 indicates the scheme for the direct use of natural resources.

Manufacturing processes based on the mining of mineral resources have increased the production of fuels and useful things. Fuel production has increased with advances in mining and mineral exploration technologies, and large amounts of thermal energy have been produced from the combustion of fossil fuels. Nuclear energy has been attracting attention as an alternative energy to prepare for the depletion of fossil fuels since the increased consumption may deplete the supply of available fossil fuels. A variety of intermediate products including chemical products, industrial materials and interchangeable parts are produced from mineral resources to manufacture the final products. High-quality chemicals are produced by carefully eliminating the impurities, and the transaction prices of chemicals are governed by their purity.

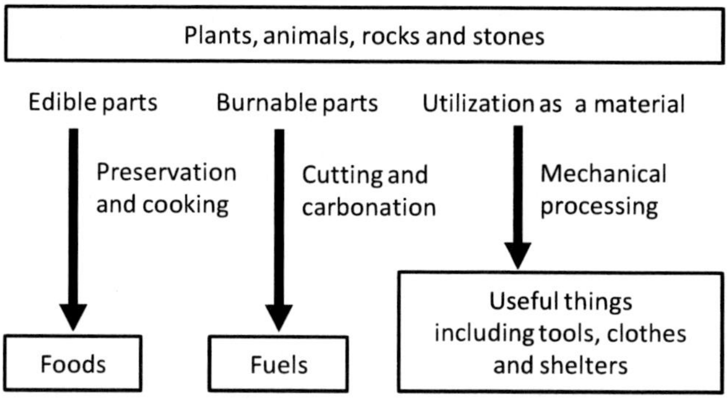


Figure 4.1. The direct use of natural resources.

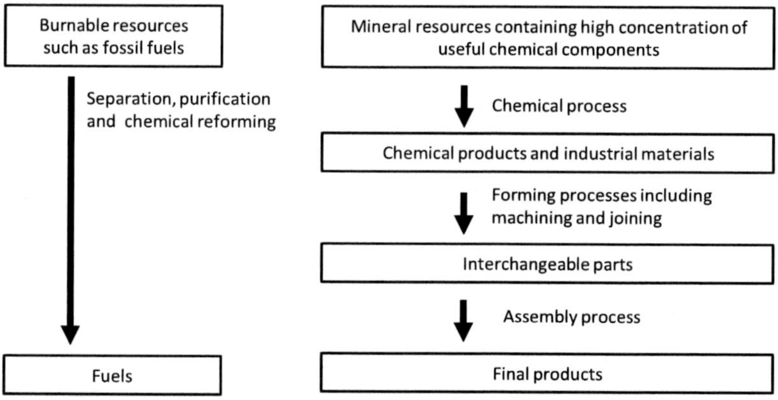


Figure 4.2. Industrial processes from mineral resources.

Industrial materials are characterized with the properties and the dimensional precision required for the production of interchangeable parts. The material properties are improved with microscopic control on various material parameters such as crystal structure, grain size, texture, and chemical compositions. Basic requirements for interchangeable parts are the dimensional precision and the performance part to meet the specifications. Casting and forging processes are efficient for shaping the metal parts, and the additional processes such as cutting and grinding further improve the precision. Some parts are welded, and the final products are manufactured by mechanically assembling the parts. Figure 4.2 shows typical industrial processes manufactured from mineral resources.

## 4.2. BIOLOGICAL RESOURCES AND FOOD PRODUCTION

A primitive method of food acquisition in hunter and gathering societies is to collect food from the surroundings by hunting animals and gathering edible plants. Unfortunately, there is a limitation in supplying enough food for the growing population. The immediate needs are to increase the availability of food for the increasing population. The solution was food production, including crop cultivation, rearing of livestock and fish farming [1, 2]. Extensive efforts have been conducted in the construction of irrigation facilities and increases in fertilizer supply because the provisions of water and fertilizer are effective for crop production. An additional requirement is to produce high-quality foods including meat production, and the productivity of meat is associated with agricultural productivity because crop production enhances the feed supply for livestock. Agricultural productivity has been further enhanced with chemical fertilizers and the mechanization of farm work, including cultivation, planting and mowing processes, as well as the technical advance in breeding crops and livestock.

### 4.2.1. Agriculture

Agricultural productivity has increased with technological progress such as improved water supply, fertilization, and cultivation techniques, and cultivation technology has advanced with the use of livestock and the development of agricultural machinery. The carrying capacity of agriculture, which is defined by the maximum population maintained by the agriculture per unit area, has been increased with advances in agricultural technology as indicated in Table 4.1 [3]. Agricultural production in slash-and-burn farming is 15 times of the hunter-gatherer society in the rainforest, and agricultural production has been promoted with advances in irrigation and fertilization. Slash-and-burn farming is the primitive form of crop cultivation where the crop is planted on burned forest. Rainfall climate contributes to water supply, and the ash is used for fertilizer. Cultivation is normally repeated for two or three years, and the place of cultivation is then moved to newly cultivated land for further cultivation because the fertilizer that is supplied by the ash is exhausted during repeated cultivations. Irrigated agriculture is a method for crop cultivation that uses the water supply from the river. Irrigated agriculture was developed in dry areas near rivers such as the Mesopotamian plain and Egypt.

**Table 4.1. Carrying capacity of agriculture [3]**

| Carrying capacity of agriculture | |
|---|---|
| Hunter-gatherer society in the rainforest | 1 |
| Slash-and-burn farming | 15 |
| Agriculture of the Middle Ages | 50 |
| Intensive tropical peasant industry in New Guinea | 125 |
| Modern intensive agriculture in Western Europe | 400 |

The lack of fertilizer was a serious problem in crop cultivation in the Middle Ages of Western Europe. As a result, the farmland was temporarily used for the grazing of livestock to fertilize the land once every few years while most livestock had to be slaughtered before winter due to the difficulty in feeding livestock during the winter. Advanced crop rotation system was developed in the 18th century to increase agricultural production, and crops of wheat, barley, turnips and clover were planted in the order. Turnips are sown for winter feed of livestock, and Rhizobium-clover symbiosis supplies fixed nitrogen in the soil. An alterative solution was adopted in Japanese cotton cultivation around the same time. Large amounts of fish fertilizer were supplied to the cotton fields after being transported by ship normally traveling several hundred kilometers or more. The artificial environment suitable for the growth of crops has been thus improved by water supply and fertilizer, and further environmental improvements for crop cultivation are in progress. Vegetables are produced in warmed greenhouses even in cold weather, and mushrooms and bean sprouts are grown in factories, in which the growing environment is automatically controlled. Hydroponic vegetables are produced in a controlled environment using mineral nutrient solutions without soil, and artificial lighting is used for cultivating plants without sunshine in some plant factories.

The development of crops having excellent taste has been achieved with the advances in breeding technology. Developed crops are prone to disease and insect damage, and pesticides are used for these problems. This is because toxic ingredients are significantly reduced in domesticated plants to improve the taste while plants contain toxic ingredients such as alkaloids to protect themselves from insects and diseases.

### 4.2.2. Livestock and Fish Farming

Meat productivity is governed by the varieties of livestock and feeding processes. White leghorn is commonly used for egg collection due to the advantages in prolific and early egg collection, and the rapid growth characteristic of broiler chicken is advantageous in meat production. Grain feeding is effective for fattening cattle to produce high-quality beef comprised of fat marbling in the muscle meat.

Feeding carp in ponds may be the origin of fish farming, and the aquaculture is advantageous in producing the fattened fish meat including oysters, eel, and prawns. Furthermore, the young salmon, artificially incubated from the eggs, are released in the river to increase the valuable fisheries resources.

## 4.3. METALS

The only available metals in the beginning of the Metal Ages were natural metals such as gold, copper and iron meteorite. Metallurgical development has expanded the range of available metals. Bronze is a hard alloy often used in the early part of the Metal Ages due to low processing temperatures. The production of iron began with the development of the high-temperature furnace. Steel is now commonly used for structural materials while various metals are used for light-weight structures and electrical devices [4, 5]. Lightweight metals such as aluminum alloys and magnesium alloys are useful for aircraft and portable devices due to the capability of constructing lightweight structures. Electric industries require a variety of materials with a wide range of electric conductivity. Electric conducting materials include copper, silver and gold, and silicon is typically used for semiconductors. In addition, ceramics and polymeric materials having high electrical resistance are used for insulators and dielectric materials.

Reductive reactions are employed for producing metallic materials since most metallic elements in the minerals are present in the forms of oxides and sulfides [6, 7]. Carbothermal reduction is a typical process to produce various metals from oxide minerals, and sulfide minerals are converted to oxides prior to the carbothermal reduction process. The electrolytic process is also applied to the production of aluminum and the purification of copper. Various metallic materials are now available with technological advances in extractive metallurgy. The machinery and construction industries have, in particular, advanced with the development of high performance steel manufactured at a low cost. Metal production has increased with the advances in manufacturing technology for extraction from abundant resources. The production of gold and silver has increased with the progress in extraction technology from crude copper, and iron production has been enhanced with the use of coke as an alternative to charcoal.

### 4.3.1. Smelting and Refining of Gold and Silver

Gold is a stable metallic element existing in nature as a simple substance. Coins and ornaments have been the major application of gold while it has recently been applied to the electric wire of integrated circuits. Gold is collected from deposits produced in riverbeds since the weathered ores have produced gold dust that settled in the bottom of a river.

Gravity concentration is used for gold dust collection.The gold dust is collected from the lower part of the sedimentation that is concentrated due to the high specific gravity. Flotation is a beneficiation method to utilize the characteristic that the minerals containing metals are hydrophobic, and the finely ground ores containing the metals and pyrites in bubbling water are selectively concentrated on the surfaces of air bubbles. The metallic particles attached to the bubbles are floated on the upper surface of the tank to be separated. The flotation is used for the beneficiation of various minerals including copper, silver and gold minerals.

Metallic solvents such as mercury and lead were used for the purification processes of gold and silver. Amalgamation produces the mercury amalgam containing gold to leave the gold after the evaporation of mercury. Since the use of mercury and lead may cause health hazards, the chemical extraction using aqueous solutions is employed in advanced processes, replacing the use of metallic solvents. Chemical extraction of gold from the ores is usually carried out with the aqueous solution of sodium cyanide (NaCN), and gold is then produced by electrolytic decomposition.

$$4\ Au + 8\ NaCN + 2H_2O + O_2 \rightarrow 4\ NaAu(CN)_2 + 4\ NaOH$$

Silver is used for electrical contacts and silver halide photography. It has also been commonly used for coins, ornaments and silverware. In silver deposits, silver minerals are typically present in forms of a simple substance and silver sulfide ($Ag_2S$) while the deposits of silver ores commonly include various metallic components such as lead, zinc, copper and gold. Advances in silver extraction from ores have been made by the cupellation process, in which silver ores are heated with the addition of lead, and the liquid lead containing silver is separated from the ores. The liquid lead phase is then oxidized to produce the lead oxide ($PbO_2$), and metallic silver is easily separated from the lead oxide.

The cupellation process was applied to the extraction of silver from crude copper. Blister copper is melted with lead at high temperatures, and the liquid metal phase is cooled slowly to separate the purified solid copper. Note that most silver is present in the metallic lead phase in this stage, and the oxidation decomposes the lead phase into lead oxide and metallic silver, and metallic silver grains are produced in the lead oxide phase. It is noteworthy that the production of gold and silver has increased with the advances in the extraction technology of precious metals contained in copper ores, and the considerable amounts of precious metals including gold and silver are currently extracted in the electrolytic refining process from crude copper, as shown in the next section.

### 4.3.2. Copper and Bronze

Today, most copper is used for electric wire. The most important alloy in ancient times was bronze for ornaments and arms, and bronze was produced from copper ores with the addition of a mineral containing tin oxide. The copper deposits usually form three layers. Copper ores in the upper layer of copper deposits contain copper oxide, copper carbonate and natural copper, and copper sulfide minerals such as chalcocite ($Cu_2S$) and covellite ($CuS$) are included in the middle layer. Today, most copper is produced from porphyry copper deposits in the lower layer of the copper deposits, which include the sulfate minerals such as bornite ($Cu_5FeS_4$) and chalcopyrite ($CuFeS_2$).

Copper content in the ores is normally within 1%, and the copper content is concentrated up to about 20 – 40% in a flotation process, in which the particles containing copper are attached to bubbles in water to be separated. Concentrated ores are then heated to separate the iron and sulfur from the copper, and the oxidation forms slag containing iron oxide and calcium sulfate separated from copper minerals. Ores concentrated with copper minerals are further oxidized to produce copper oxides by removing sulfur, and the carbothermal reduction is followed to prepare the crude copper of 99% purity.

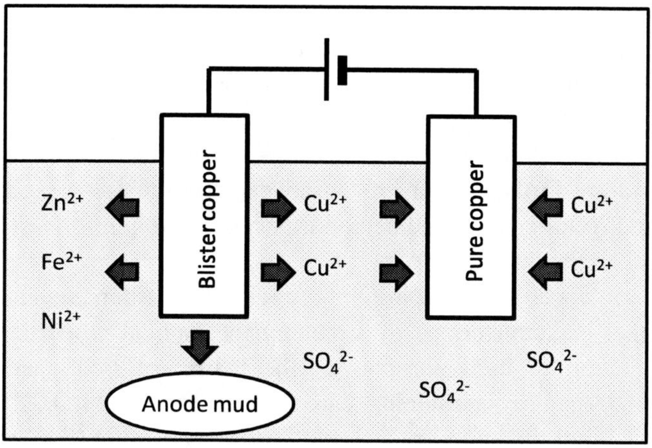


Figure 4.3. Electrolytic refining of copper.

The crude copper is further purified in the electrolytic refining process, in which electrolysis is carried out in an aqueous solution of copper sulfate and sulfuric acid. As shown in Figure 4.3, copper ions dissolved from the anode consisting of a crude copper plate are deposited on the cathode plate of pure copper, and the pure copper of 99.99% or more is produced. Impurities such as gold, silver, selenium and silicate are precipitated under the anode as an anode mud, whereas some elements such as iron, nickel and zinc remain in the aqueous solution. As a result, valuable metallic elements including gold and silver are condensed in the bottom of the reaction container.

### 4.3.3. Iron and Steel

Iron ores are abundantly available all over the world, and the mechanical properties of steel are advantageous in their application to mechanical parts. Iron is basically produced with the carbon reduction of iron ores, and the reductive reaction is promoted at high temperatures. Advances in furnace technology has therefore increased iron production and improved the quality of iron products.

Wrought iron is the iron product processed at relatively low temperatures, and the iron ores are reduced with charcoal to produce the spongy iron that is the mixture of porous iron and residual silicates. Most of the residual silicates are eliminated during the hot-forging process that is performed to beat out the silicate from the spongy iron to produce the wrought iron. Wrought iron has a composite structure containing a small amount of residual silicate dispersed in a matrix of iron, and the material is reinforced with the fibrous silicate particles produced during the hot-forging process.

Pig iron is a solidified molten iron, and the molten iron is produced in a high-temperature furnace. Cast iron, produced from the re-melted pig iron, is characterizedby hard and brittle behavior because it contains a large amount of carbon (about 4 %).

Steel is produced from pig iron by reducing the carbon content to less than 2%. The steel is characterized by excellent mechanical properties due to the fine precipitation of hard particles in the matrix of iron. Carbon steel is basically an iron alloy containing carbon in the range of 0.02 to 2%. The materials are reinforced with the fine particles of cementite ($Fe_3C$) precipitated in the iron matrix. The mechanical properties of carbon steel are further improved with heat treatments such as quenching and tempering, and the composite structure of hard precipitates in the iron matrix is optimized by the heat treatment to improve its performance. Mechanical properties and corrosion resistance of carbon steels are further improved with alloy steels, in which various elements are added to improve the material properties.

The pig iron is produced from iron ores with a reductive reaction at high temperatures. The powerful blast mechanism has increased the furnace temperature to produce the molten iron. It is important to note that the melting temperature of pig iron is considerably lower than the pure iron due to the dissolution of carbon around 4%. Pig iron had already been produced in the Warring States Period (476 BC – 221 BC) in China, and the bellows driven by manpower produced the powerful blast mechanism for achieving high temperatures. In Western Europe, the production of pig iron began in the 15th century using charcoal, and the bellows were driven by water wheels. The biggest problem in mass production of iron at the time was the huge consumption of charcoal, leading to the possible extinction of forests. The use of coal as a substitute for charcoal for blast furnaces requires the elimination of the sulfur contained in coal because the contamination of sulfur degrades the mechanical properties of steel. The solution was the coking process, and the coke was produced with the carbonization of coal. Pig iron production using coke was started around 1270 in China, and the first production in the Western Europe was made by Abraham Darby in 1709.

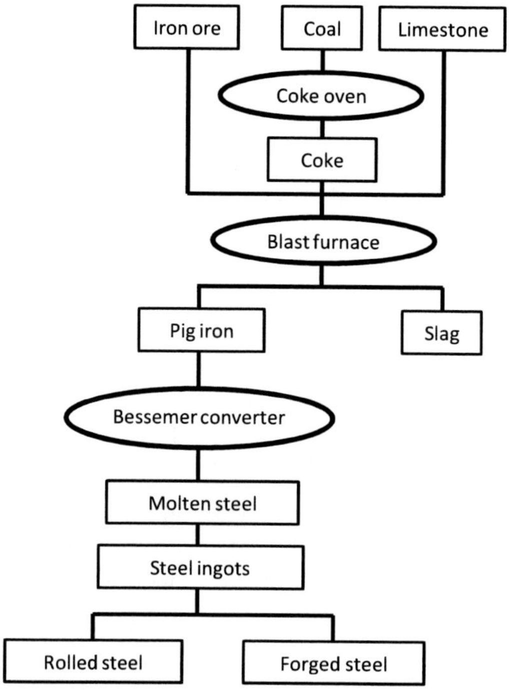


Figure 4.4. Modern steelmaking processes.

Steel production from pig iron requires the elimination of excess carbon, and the residual carbon content dominates the mechanical properties of steel. Note that most structural steel contains a small amount of carbon ranging from 0.1 to 0.6 %, and the carbon contents of hard steel such as tool steels are in the range of 0.6 to 1.4% [4]. Successful elimination of the excess carbon was made possible by the paddling method using a reverberatory furnace, which was patented by Henry Court in 1784, and the excess carbon is gradually removed by stirring the molten iron with rods. Considerable progress was made by the invention of the Bessemer converter developed by Henry Bessemer in 1856. In the Bessemer converter, air is blown into the molten iron to promote the violent oxidation reaction accompanied with heat generation, and a rapid decrease in excess carbon occurs.

Steel products are machined and joined together to make the final products, and heat treatments are often conducted for improving their performance. In addition, the surface hardening treatment of steel is typically carried out with carburizing, and the materials are strengthened with heat treatments such as quenching and tempering. In recent years, the excess carbon in the pig iron, produced in the blast furnace, is generally reduced in the advanced converter in which oxygen is blown. Figure 4.4 shows the typical process for modern steelmaking.

### 4.3.4. Aluminum and the Related Metals

The varieties of available metallic materials have increased with the advance in extractive metallurgy. Metallic materials such as bronze and steel have been produced in carbothermal reduction processes, and the electrolytic process is capable of producing base metals such as aluminum. Base metals are, in general, characterized by light-weight, and the light-weight equipment including airplanes have been developed with the advances in light-weight materials.

Aluminum alloys have been commonly applied to airplanes, automobiles and the high-voltage electric power lines. The major ore for producing aluminum is bauxite, which contains the minerals of aluminum hydroxides such as gibbsite, $Al(OH)_3$, boehmite, $\gamma$-AlO(OH) and diaspore, $\alpha$-AlO(OH). Aluminum is chemically extracted from the bauxite by dissolving it in a sodium hydroxide aqua solution at elevated temperatures, and aluminum hydroxide, precipitated during the cooling process, is converted to aluminum oxide by calcinations. Aluminum had been produced in an expensive chemical reduction process using metallic sodium or potassium for reducing agents because the carbothermal reduction process of aluminum oxide could not be applied. The aluminum metal is now produced by the electrolytic process, in which cryolite ($Na_3AlF_6$) is used for the electrolyte.

Magnesium alloys having lower densities than aluminum alloys are used for the light-weight parts in automobiles and portable electric devices. The magnesium metal is produced by either the electrolysis of molten $MgCl_2$ or the chemical reduction with ferrosilicon. In the electrolysis process, $MgCl_2$ is produced from the chemical reaction of MgO, C and $Cl_2$ gas, and the molten $MgCl_2$ is then electrolyzed around 700°C to produce magnesium metal while generating the by-product of $Cl_2$ gas. The chemical reduction of MgO with the addition of ferrosilicon (Fe-Si alloy) is conducted at around 1200°C in a vacuum to generate magnesium vapor, which is to be deposited on the cold parts of the reaction vessel.

Titanium exhibits an excellent corrosion resistance, and the biological stability of titanium alloys is applied to implant materials. Metallic titanium is produced by the chemical reduction of titanium tetrachloride ($TiCl_4$) gas with liquid magnesium at 800°C, and titanium tetrachloride is produced from ilumenite ($FeTiO_3$) reacted with carbon and chlorine gas at 900°C.

$$2\ FeTiO_3 + 7\ Cl_2 + 6\ C \rightarrow 2\ TiCl_4 + 2\ FeCl_3 + 6\ CO$$

$$2Mg + TiCl_4 \rightarrow 2MgCl_2 + Ti$$

Most silicon is used for aluminum-silicon alloys and semiconductor devices. Aluminum-silicon alloys are produced from metallurgical-grade silicon, which is produced by carbon reduction of silica in an electric arc furnace using carbon electrodes. Semiconductor devices require further purification, and metallurgical-grade silicon is purified in the form of a gaseous state such as $SiH_4$, $SiHCl_3$ and $SiCl_4$ to produce silicon crystals. Solar grade silicon typically requires higher purity than 99.9999% (6N), and semiconductor grade requires much higher purity than 99.999999999% (11N) to be provided in the form of single crystals having an extremely low concentration of lattice defects.

## 4.4. CHEMICALS

The chemical industry has developed with the advances in processing basic chemicals such as sulfuric acid, soda and ammonia [8-10]. In the textile industry that developed in the era of the Industrial Revolution, the conventional cloth bleaching process was improved by the invention of bleaching power and the advanced manufacturing process of sulfuric acid. In addition, the development of efficient processes in the soda industry has enhanced the productivities of soap and glass.

The chemical synthesis of nitrogen fertilizer enhanced agricultural production, and the productivity of ammonia was improved with the development of the Haber-Bosch process. Chemical processes have evolved with the development of innovative processes using abundant natural resources to reduce the environmental impacts while the incremental improvements have been carried out.

### 4.4.1. Sulfuric Acid

Sulfuric acid is used for the production of various chemicals, including chemical fertilizers and laundry detergent, and dilute sulfuric acid is used for the lead-acid battery electrolyte. Sulfuric acid was produced with the dry distillation of iron sulfate hydrate ($FeSO_4 \cdot 7H_2O$) by Geber (Jābir ibn Hayyān), an Islamic alchemist in the eighth century.

The discovery of effective oxidizing agents to produce sulfur trioxide ($SO_3$) from sulfur dioxide ($SO_2$) has promoted sulfuric acid production from sulfur. Note that sulfur trioxide reacts with water to produce sulfuric acid, and sulfur dioxide is easily produced by the oxidation of sulfur.

$$S + O_2 \rightarrow SO_2$$

$$H_2O + SO_3 \rightarrow H_2SO_4$$

The oxidation agent is needed in the oxidation step of sulfur dioxide to produce sulfur trioxide, and the process innovation has been made by the development of the oxidizing agent to produce the purified sulfuric acid. The first industrial oxidizing agent was saltpeter ($KNO_3$), and the product contains a considerable amount of nitric acid because nitrogen dioxide is generated by the decomposition of potassium nitrate at elevated temperatures, and nitrogen dioxide oxidizes sulfur dioxide as follows.

$$NO_2 + SO_2 \rightarrow SO_3 + NO$$

The chemical stability is important for the reaction vessel since saltpeter has a strong oxidization ability and sulfuric acid exhibits strong acidity. Glass containers were used for the vessel in 1736 while large reaction vessels were required for an increase in production.

John Roebuck developed the lead-chamber process in 1746, and the additional improvements in the lead-chamber process continued, with the recovery of nitrogen oxide as by-products in 1827 and the separation of nitric acid in 1859.

A great advance was made by the contact process that uses a vanadium catalyst developed in 1915, and the contact process has replaced the conventional process for sulfuric acid production.

**Table 4.2. Progress in sulfuric acid production**

| Year | Progress |
|---|---|
| 8th Century | Dry distillation of $FeSO_4 \cdot 7H_2O$ |
| 1736 | Oxidation of $SO_2$ by $KNO_3$ |
| 1915 | Contact process for the oxidization of $SO_2$ with catalyst of $V_2O_5$ |

$$SO_2 + O_2 \rightarrow SO_3$$

This process uses a solid catalyst of $V_2O_5$ for the oxidation of sulfur dioxide to produce sulfuric acid of high concentration while containing lower amounts of impurity. In recent processes, sulfuric acid is produced from various sulfur sources such as iron sulfide, the desulfurization of petroleum and the roasting gas of sulfide ores. The progress in sulfuric acid production is summarized in Table 4.2.

## 4.4.2. Alkali and Soda Ashes

A large amount of alkali, including baking soda (sodium hydrogen carbonate, $NaHCO_3$), soda ash (sodium carbonate anhydride, $Na_2CO_3$) and caustic soda (sodium hydroxide, NaOH), is used for the manufacture of glass and soap, and the alkali compounds are chemically interchangeable. Soda ash is produced with heating the baking soda, and caustic soda is produced from the reaction of soda ash and calcium hydrate in an aqueous solution.

$$2\ NaHCO_3 \rightarrow Na_2CO_3 + CO_2 + H_2O$$

$$Na_2CO_3 + Ca(OH)_2 \rightarrow 2\ NaOH + CaCO_3$$

Natron and wood ash are historically important alkali resources. Natron is a natural mixture containing sodium carbonate decahydrate ($Na_2CO_3 \cdot 10H_2O$) sometimes found in arid environments, and wood ash contains a large amount of potassium. Although the origin of glass is unclear, the ancient glass, unearthed in Egypt and the West Asia, has revealed that the ancient glass has been produced from sand and natron. The origin of soap is also unclear. Soap was produced from sheep fat and wood ash around AD 130 in Gallia. The industrial production of soap started around the eighth century in the Southern Europe. Today, glass is prepared from the mixture of limestone (calcium carbonate, $CaCO_3$), feldspar, soda ash and silica sand at high temperatures, and soap is prepared from caustic soda reacting with vegetable oils or animal fats. Progress in the manufacturing process of soda has thus contributed to the increased production of glass and soap.

The Leblanc process is the first mass production process of soda ash that has been commercialized while serious problems are caused by the harmful by-products of hydrogen chloride and calcium sulfide.

The problems were solved by the development of Solvay process because the by-product is harmless calcium chloride. A further advance was made by the chlor-alkali process, which is the electrolysis of brine to produce a valuable product of chlorine gas in addition to the production of sodium hydroxide. Therefore, the major advance in the process may be characterized by the reduction of the worthless by-products with an increase in the valuable products. The progress in soda production is summarized in Table 4.3.

**Table 4.3. Progress in soda production**

| Year | Progress |
|---|---|
| 1791 | Leblanc process (Soda ash industry to produce $Na_2CO_3$, HCl and CaS) |
| 1861 | Solvay process (Soda ash industry to produce $Na_2CO_3$ and $CaCl_2$) |
| 1892 | Chlor-alkali process (Electrolytic soda industry to produce NaOH, $Cl_2$ and $H_2$) |

#### *4.4.2.1. Leblanc Process*

Baking soda and soda ash had been provided by the mineral resources consisting of sodium carbonate and sodium hydrogen carbonate. The Leblanc process successfully manufactured soda from rock salt. In the first step, rock salt is heated with sulfuric acid to produce sodium sulfate and hydrogen chloride.

$$2\ NaCl + H_2SO_4 \rightarrow Na_2SO_4 + 2\ HCl$$

In the second step, the mixture of sodium sulfate, limestone and coal is heated to produce the mixture of calcium sulfide and sodium carbonate.

$$Na_2SO_4 + CaCO_3 + 2C \rightarrow Na_2CO_3 + CaS + 2\ CO_2$$

Sodium carbonate is separated from the product by washing it with water because sodium carbonate is the only product dissolvable in water. Soda production by the Leblanc process was started in 1791, and a large amount of soda was produced in the 19th century. The problem with this process is air pollution due to the released chemical substances, such as hydrogen chloride and hydrogen sulfide. This is because hydrogen chloride is released into the atmosphere and the hydrogen sulfide is generated with the reaction of calcium sulfide with water.

#### *4.4.2.2. Solvay Process*

The ammonia soda process or Solvay process was industrialized by Ernest Solvay in 1861. The baking soda is precipitated from the solution when carbon dioxide gas flows into an aqueous solution of saturated sodium chloride in which ammonia is filled.

$$NaCl + H_2O + NH_3 + CO_2 \rightarrow NH_4Cl + NaHCO_3$$

In the process, carbon dioxide is supplied from the thermal decomposition of limestone, and ammonium chloride is to be reacted with slaked lime to regenerate ammonia.

$$CaCO_3 \rightarrow CaO + CO_2$$

$$Ca(OH)_2 + 2\ NH_4Cl \rightarrow CaCl_2 + 2\ H_2O + 2\ NH_3$$

The summarized reaction process of the Solvay process may be expressed as the production of calcium chloride and soda ash from salt and limestone with no consumption of ammonia.

$$CaCO_3 + 2\ NaCl \rightarrow CaCl_2 + Na_2CO_3$$

In this process, the by-product of calcium chloride is harmless in comparison with the by-product of hydrogen chloride and calcium sulfide in the Leblanc process.

#### *4.4.2.3. Chlor-Alkali Process*

The Chlor-alkali process is basically the electrolysis of brine to produce chlorine and caustic soda. Industrial production utilizing this process began in 1892. Large quantities of chlorine, produced by the electrolysis of brine, are now consumed in the manufacture of various chemicals including polyvinyl chloride and hydrochloric acid. In the electrolysis of brine, chlorine gas is generated from the positive electrode or anode, and hydrogen gas is normally generated from the negative electrode or cathode. In chlor-alkali process, concentrated sodium hydroxide is collected in the vicinity of the negative electrode or cathode, and three variations are known to produce sodium hydroxide in the electrolysis of brine: the diaphragm-cell process, the mercury-cell process and the membrane-cell process.

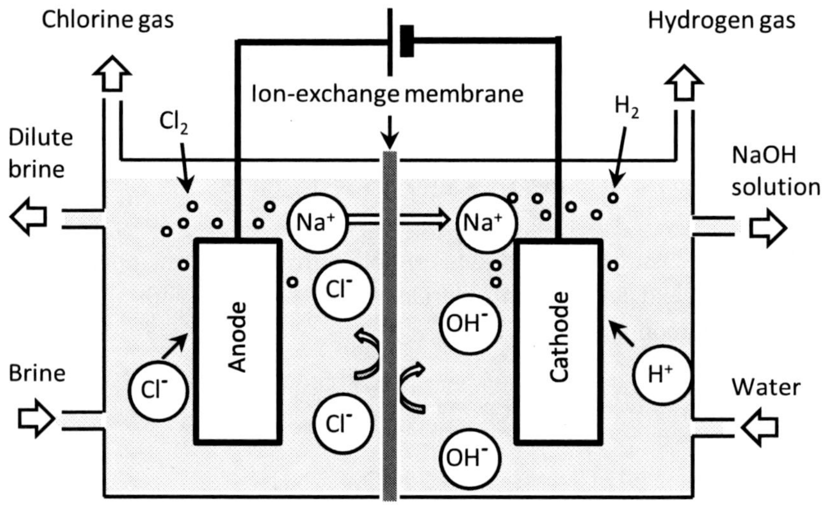


Figure 4.5. Membrane-cell process to produce soda and chlorine.

The diaphragm-cell process was developed to retrieve a high concentration of sodium hydroxide in the vicinity of the negative electrode, and the diaphragm of asbestos fiber is provided as a separator between the negative electrode and the electrolyte of salt water to obtain the sodium hydroxide containing a small amount of impurity salt. High purity sodium hydroxide is produced in the mercury-cell process because sodium amalgam is formed on the mercury electrode, and sodium hydroxide is taken out by the reaction of the sodium amalgam with water. A major concern of the process is the use of the toxic substance of mercury, and further advances were made by the chlor-alkali process to replace the toxic substance with an ion-exchange membrane for the diaphragm. Figure 4.5 illustrates the chlor-alkali membrane-cell process, in which the aqueous solution of sodium hydroxide is taken out without containing rock salt because the ion-selective membrane allows the sodium ions to freely flow across while preventing chlorine ions from diffusing across.

## 4.4.3. Ammonia Production

In the late 19th century, nitratine ($NaNO_3$) was used for nitrogen fertilizer. A major concern was the food crisis due to the possible exhaustion of nitratine resources. Therefore, the advanced processes for nitrogen fertilizer have been extensively explored, and the Haber-Bosch process was successfully established.

Ammonia is an important chemical substance for the production of nitrogen fertilizer such as ammonium sulfate and urea, and nitric acid is produced by the oxidation of ammonia. It is important to note that the oxidation process for ammonia was developed by Friedrich Wilhelm Ostwald in 1902. In the Ostwald process, ammonia is oxidized to form NO in the presence of Pt catalyst at high temperature, and nitric acid is produced from $NO_2$ that is formed during the cooling process of NO.

### *4.4.3.1. Ammonia Production from Nitrogen in Air*

Two processes for fixing air nitrogen have been developed as a candidate of nitrogen fertilizer for an alternative to nitratine. One is to fix air nitrogen in the form of calcium cyanamid ($CaCN_2$) by the reaction between calcium carbide and nitrogen.This process was industrialized in 1904. The second is to obtain nitrate from nitrogen oxide that is produced by an arc discharge in the air. This process was industrialized in 1905. Both manufacturing processes require large amounts of electric power because the former produces calcium carbide from a mixture of coke and lime using a high temperature reaction around 2000°C in an electric furnace, and the latter uses electric power for arc discharge.

Calcium cyanamid is produced by the reaction of calcium carbide and nitrogen, and calcium carbide is produced by the carbon reduction of calcium oxide that is generated in the thermal decomposition of limestone.

$$CaO + 3\,C \rightarrow CaC_2 + 2\,CO$$

$$CaC_2 + N_2 \rightarrow CaCN_2 + C$$

Calcium cyanamid is effective as a fertilizer due to ammonia generation by the reaction with water.

$$CaCN_2 + 3\,H_2O \rightarrow 2\,NH_3 + CaCO_3$$

NO is formed by the high temperature reaction in the arc discharge between nitrogen and oxygen in the air. As the temperature decreases, NO reacts with oxygen to form $NO_2$. Nitric acid is then produced from $NO_2$ being absorbed in water.

$$3\ NO_2 + H_2O \rightarrow 2\ HNO_3 + NO$$

#### *4.4.3.2. Haber-Bosch Process*

Le Chatelier's principle for chemical equilibrium was published in 1884. The chemical equilibrium predicted the possible conditions for ammonia production from nitrogen in air.

$$N_2 + 3\ H_2 \rightarrow 2\ NH_3 + 92.2\ kJ$$

Analysis of the equilibrium has revealed that a higher concentration of ammonia is achieved at higher pressures and lower temperatures. In the production of ammonia by the reaction of hydrogen and nitrogen, the major technical problems were (i) to develop the material suitable for a high-pressure vessel having no degradation under the exposure to hot hydrogen, (ii) to develop the catalyst affordable to lower the reaction temperature, (iii) to produce hydrogen and nitrogen gases for raw materials. In the Haber-Bosch process, the ammonia synthesis was achieved at the temperature of 500°C under a pressure of 200 atm.

The development includes (i) the reaction tube having a double-tube structure that combines an outer steel tube of high strength and an inner tube of chrome-vanadium steel having low-carbon content to reduce the chemical reactivity to hot hydrogen, (ii) an advanced catalyst system consisting of the aluminum oxide, iron oxide and potassium oxide, and (iii) the low cost production of a gas mixture of nitrogen and hydrogen.

Low cost production of the gas mixture was achieved in a two-step process. The first step is the mixed gas production of nitrogen, hydrogen and carbon dioxide by reacting steam with carbon monoxide in the producer gas, and the second step is to eliminate carbon dioxide gas from the mixture by absorbing it in water with pressurizing the gas mixture. Industrial production was started in 1913, and the progress in the fixing process for air nitrogen is summarized in Table 4.4.

**Table 4.4. Progress in fixing process for air nitrogen**

| Year | Progress |
|---|---|
| 1904 | Production of calcium cyanamid |
| 1905 | Arc discharge in the air to produce nitrogen oxide |
| 1913 | Ammonia production by the Haber-Bosch process |

## 4.5. Mechanical Parts and Assembly Process

The quality and productivity of industrial products in the Middle Ages was governed by the skill of the craftsmen's handiwork, and the demand for industrial products has increased with economic development. Productivities in machining and assembly processes have been enhanced with the division of labor, mechanization and process automation, and large scale production is inevitable for recovering the increased fixed cost due to the investment in mass production facilities.

A large amount of energy is consumed in the large production facilities and high productivity is achieved by reducing the number of factory workers.

### 4.5.1. Handicraft

Industrial products originated from crafts that were manufactured by craftsmen, and the quality and productivity were governed by the skill of craftsmen's handiwork. This was the primary mode of production in the Middle Ages. The technical skill was enhanced with proficiency developed over a long period of time.

The quality of products was greatly influenced by workmanship, and the skill was handed down through the apprenticeship. It was therefore difficult to increase production in a short period of time because production was governed by the number of craftsmen having technical skills acquired by work experience over a long period of time.

### 4.5.2. Division of Labor

The division of labor enhances productivity, as found by Adam Smith [11]. The manufacturing work in the artisanal manufacturing process is divided into simple tasks comprised of standardized procedures, and each worker, engaged in the particular process to repeat the routine tasks, becomes proficient with short-term training due to the simple task. As a result, the workers become proficient within a short time period to produce a number of products with uniform quality, and mass production of industrial products has been achieved.

### 4.5.3. Mechanization

Further improvements in productivity have been made through mechanization, which has completely changed the working process. Machinery has replaced manual labor, and the skill required for operators is the manipulation of the machines, instead of manipulating the hand tools in handicraft. As a result, the impact of mechanization has been to hire machine operators and to fire skilled artisans. Textile machinery has developed during the early stages of the industrial revolution. The development of spinning machines and looms has significantly increased textile production.

Water wheels were used as the major power sources of mechanization in the Middle Ages while the locations for the machinery were limited due to the availability of natural power sources. The restrictions on the plant location were eliminated with advanced power sources such as steam engines, gas engines and electric motors. Production has increased in the factories equipped with the advanced power sources.

Productivity in the assembly industries has greatly advanced with the provision of interchangeable components, as well as the progress in the mechanization of part production and assembly processes. Interchangeable mechanical parts are required for the dimensional variations limited within allowable range, and the parts are produced with quality-controlled materials having standardized dimensions. Metal parts are, in general, produced by casting and forging processes followed by cutting and grinding. Processing machinery such as lathes and grinding machines, as well as the development of dimensional inspection equipment, has contributed to the production of interchangeable parts. The development in precision machinery such as the lathe and milling machine has produced cylinders and pistons for steam engines, and the boring machine invented by John Wilkinson has manufactured the precise shape of cylinders to accomodate James Watt's steam engines. Furthermore, the production of interchangeable parts has resulted in the development of assembly industries such as guns, sewing machines, typewriters, bicycles and automobiles [12].

### 4.5.4. Automation

Further advancements were made with the automation process. The production speed was greatly enhanced with automated machines, and the central task for workers became the monitoring of the mass production facilities. Consequently, enormous investments have been made to mechanize the assembly industry, including the textile industry, the machinery industry and the automotive industry [13]. The investment is recovered from the profit earned by the large amount of production consuming a large amount of energy supplied to the facilities to reduce the number of factory workers.

Individual machine operators are unnecessary for automated production facilities. The major tasks for the workers are to monitor and control the operation. Industrial production in the 20th century has advanced with unattended manufacturing facilities, and the mass production technology has been applied to a variety of industrial production processes although significant labor is still required in the current assembly processes such as the automotive assembly, the electrical applicance assembly and the sewing process of clothes.

Automated production has greatly progressed in chemical industries because the chemical synthesis is conducted in an unattended reaction vessel. The process control is important for chemical production, and the major task for operators in large-scale plants, including chemical plants, steel industries, cement industries and power plants, is to monitor the operation. However, the ability to make adequate judgments is required on the basis of the detailed knowledge and a complete understanding of the equipment in emergency situations such as unexpected accidents in chemical plants and nuclear power plants.

## REFERENCES

[1] Sauer, C. O., *Agricultural Origins and Dispersals*, American Geographical Society, NY, 1952.

[2] Isaac, E., *Geography of Domestication*, Prentice-Hall, NJ, 1970.

[3] Southwood, R., *The Story of Life*, Oxford University Press, Oxford, 2004.

[4] Callister, Jr., W. D. and Rethwisch, D. G., *Materials Science and Engineering: An Introduction*, Wiley, NY, 2006.

[5] Ashby, M. F. and Jones, D. R. H., *Engineering Materials 2*, Pergamon Press, Oxford, 1986.

[6] Gilchrist, J.D., *Extraction Metallurgy*, Pergamon Press, Oxford, 1989.

[7] Rosenqvist, T., *Principles of Extractive Metallurgy*, Tapir Academic Press, Trondheim, 2004.

[8] Haber, L. F., *The Chemical Industry During the Nineteenth Century*, Oxford University Press, Oxford, 1958.

[9] Haber, L. F., *The Chemical Industry 1900-1930*, Oxford University Press, Oxford, 1971.

[10] Büchel, K. H., Moretto, H.-H., Woditsch, P., *Industrial Inorganic Chemistry*, Wiley-VCH, Weinhein, 2000.

[11] Smith, A., *Inquiry into the Nature and Causes of the Wealth of Nations*, Strahan and Cadell, London, 1776.

[12] Rolt, L. C. T., *Tools for the Job, A Short History of Machine Tools*, Batsford, London, 1965.

[13] Hounshell, D. A., *From the American System to Mass Production, 1800–1932*, Johns Hopkins University Press, Baltimore, MD, 1984.

*Chapter 5*

# TECHNOLOGICAL PROGRESS

Immediate needs are the minimum requirements for human survival to be satisfied with the provision of sufficient amounts of agricultural and industrial products necessary for life. The improvements in the manufacturing process are important for enhancing productivity. Additional requirements are to supply the high-quality products for enhancing well-being, and that needs are satisfied at higher levels by supplying higher-quality products, such as delicious meals, comfortable clothes and comfortable living environments. High-quality products are primarily developed with incremental improvements in existing technologies. The development of advanced technologies is driven by creative ingenuity and the application of scientific knowledge. Additional needs include the enhancement of convenience and the developments in transportation and communication technologies have greatly contributed to the convenience in life. Convenient functions are mostly produced by the new combinations of existing technologies, and the excellent ingenuity plays an important role in inventive activities [1, 2].

Scientific knowledge is based on the discoveries of scientific facts and phenomena, and the regularity may be induced from the accumulation of similar facts and phenomena [3]. The discovery of regularity is originally proposed as a hypothesis that needs verification, and the verified hypothesis is regarded as scientific law. Independent scientific laws may be deduced from the assumption of simple principles, and the predictions theoretically deduced from the principles are compared with scientific facts. Once the theoretical framework is established, the theoretical analyses become useful for solving various engineering problems.

Valuable discoveries of scientific facts and phenomena have directly advanced the performance of industrial products. Some of the great breakthroughs have been promoted with accidental discoveries. The invention of dynamite is associated with the discovery that diatomaceous earth has a stabilizing effect for nitroglycerin, and the invention of dynamite has greatly enhanced the performance of explosives. Silver halide photography has advanced with the discovery that the latent image is developed by exposure to mercury vapor, and the invention of the electromagnet is associated with the discovery of electromagnetic induction. The law of isochronism of the simple pendulum, discovered by Galileo Galilei, was later applied to the invention of the pendulum clock by Christiaan Huygens in 1656. The laws of chemical equilibrium, proposed by Le Châtelier in 1884, were applied to the prediction of ammonia synthesis conditions from nitrogen in air in 1901. The development of wireless technology **is associated with the Maxwell's theory** that has revealed the presence of electromagnetic waves, and the theoretical progress in atomic physics has resulted in the development of atomic bombs and nuclear reactors. In addition, the advance in engineering materials and medical technology is closely associated with the accidental discoveries of scientific facts [4, 5]. The deep understanding of scientific theories is thus useful for advancing the technologies. The three stages of scientific knowledge are summarized in Figure 5.1.

Steam engines had been incrementally improved by the efforts of Thomas Savery, Thomas Newcomen and James Watt, and further progress in the steam engines led to the evolution in the transportation systems such as steamboats and steam locomotives [6].

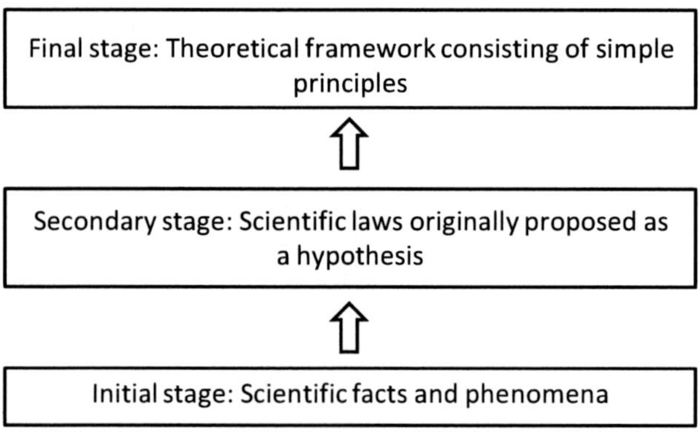


Figure 5.1. Three stages in scientific knowledge.

Compact steam engines with high output power were developed for steam locomotives by employing high steam pressure. Electric motors are used in a variety of electrical products, including electric fans, washing machines and vacuum cleaners. The application has been promoted with the creative ingenuity of combining the existing technologies of mechanical components with electric motors.

In addition, the integration of information and communication technologies has increased the convenience through a computer network, and the business models using the Internet and e-mail have grown substantially in the early 21st century. Therefore, important factors in technological progress for achieving the comfortable and convenient lifestyle may be summarized as (i) the scientific discoveries and their application, (ii) establishing the theoretical framework and its application and (iii) the incremental improvements of existing technologies.

The contribution of these factors depends on the developmental stage in science and technology. The primary stage in technological development is promoted with the direct application of scientific knowledge, and technological advances have been directly promoted with the valuable discoveries.

The secondary stage is the application of the theoretical framework, and innovative products are theoretically predicted. The final stage is to improve the conventional technology, and incremental improvements are conducted for advancing the performance of products while reducing the production cost. The inventing ingenuity plays an important role in advancing the technologies to meet the customer needs.

The theoretical framework has greatly promoted the technological progress in electric and nuclear technology. In the 19th century, the nature of electricity and magnetism was intensively explored since the invention of the voltaic pile, and the scientific knowledge was formulated in electromagnetism. The application of electromagnetism began in the late 19th century, and innovative products, including electric power generators and radio broadcasting, have been developed. In addition, numerous outstanding inventions such as silver-halide photography and internal combustion engines were promoted with ingenuity of the great inventors in the 19th century. In the early 20th century, intensive study was conducted in the field of atomic physics, and the discovery of nuclear fission triggered the development of innovative products such as nuclear reactors and atomic bombs. The contribution of scientific discovery has been significant in the fields of chemical processes, materials science, and pharmaceutical technology, and valuable discoveries have directly contributed to the technological development.

Once the primitive technology is developed, the technological progress is promoted with the incremental improvements of existing technologies. Therefore, technology is originally initiated with the great application of scientific facts and theories, and further advances are promoted with inventing ingenuity. Note that the appropriate activities to effectively promote the technological progress depend on the evolutional stage of individual technologies.

## 5.1. Progress in Mechanical Technologies

The main components of traditional machinery, in which the mechanical power is supplied with human power, animal power, hydropower and wind power, are composed of the power transmission mechanisms combining a variety of mechanical elements such as bearings, gears and shafts. The intended function is exerted through the adequate combination of mechanical components.

The basic requirements for the mechanical elements are to withstand high contact stresses having excellent wear resistance. In addition, low friction is required for the parts attached to the shaft in the bearing system. The gear mechanism is used for converting the direction and speed in rotary motion, and the conversion between rotary and reciprocating motions is conducted with the crank and cam mechanisms.

The combination of mechanical elements had resulted in the development of mechanical clocks and automatic dolls driven by the mechanical energy stored in the mainspring. Flour mills were driven by water wheels and windmills in the Middle Ages. Technology that was developed in the Middle Ages was based on the scientific knowledge empirically known, and creative ingenuity has played an important role in advancing the technology. Modern industry has developed with the technological progress in power sources such as steam engines, internal combustion engines and electric motors, and technical progress is associated with advances in structural materials and the control technology. Most of the mechanical technologies are based on the **combination of existing technologies modified to meet the customer's needs,** and the products have been incrementally improved towards the optimal design.

### 5.1.1. Steam Engines

In 1643, a vacuum was discovered by Evangelista Torricelli, who filled mercury in a glass tube closed at one end and measured the height of the mercury. The height was constant at about 76 cm, and the vacuum was formed on the top. Otto von Guericke conducted the famous experiment in 1657 to measure the power of a vacuum. This experiment is known as the Magdeburg hemispheres. In the experiment, the vacuum was produced by extracting air from two metallic hemispheres combined together, and the vacuum power was evaluated with the number of horses to pull out the hemisphere. The experiment revealed the strong power of the vacuum because the hemispheres could not be separated by the power of sixteen horses.

Thomas Savery developed the Miner's Friend or a drainage pump system using a vacuum in 1698. The pump system was composed of a cold water tank, a boiler, a vessel, valves and pipes. The vessel was initially filled with steam, and the vacuum was produced in the vessel by injecting cold water from the water tank into the vessel to condense the steam. The drainage was sucked up into the vacuum vessel through the drainage pipe, and the drainage was extruded upward through another drainage pipe with steam pressure. This was operated by opening and closing the valves. The automated valve operation was invented by Humphrey Potter in 1713.

A piston was installed in a vessel cylinder of the steam engine developed by Thomas Newcomen in 1712, and the piston was allowed to exercise up and down by creating a vacuum in a space at the bottom of the piston in the cylinder. A vacuum is produced by injecting water into the cylinder which has been filled with steam in advance supplied from the boiler. The drawback of Newcomen's engine was low thermal efficiency, resulting from the enormous consumption of thermal energy for heating and cooling the cylinder. This is because the water spray in the cylinder reduces the cylinder temperature and the refilling of steam to the cylinder consumes the additional thermal energy for heating the cylinder. In 1776, James Watt successfully reduced the heat loss by attaching a separate condenser where the cooling and heating operations are performed. The improved efficiency of Watt's steam engine results from the smaller heat capacity of the condenser than the huge cylinder, as described in the Watt's first patent in 1769. The creative ingenuity has made incremental improvements in the steam engine technology while the discovery of scientific knowledge on vacuums has initiated the application of vacuums to steam engines, as summarized in Table 5.1.

**Table 5.1. Great achievements in the development of steam engines**

| Year | Achievements (Contributor) |
|---|---|
| 1643 | Discovery of vacuum (Evangelista Torricelli) |
| 1657 | Magdeburg hemispheres to measure the power of vacuum (Otto von Guericke) |
| 1698 | Drainage pump system using vacuum (Thomas Savery) |
| 1712 | Development of reciprocating steam engines (Thomas Newcomen) |
| 1769 | Watt's patent to install the condenser in reciprocating steam engines (James Watt) |
| 1776 | Watt's first steam engine installed in commercial enterprises (James Watt) |
| 1779 | Development of high pressure steam engines (Richard Trevithick) |
| 1801 | Demonstration of steam locomotive (Richard Trevithick) |
| 1825 | Business operation of steam locomotive (George Stephenson) |

### 5.1.2. High-Pressure Steam Engines and Internal Combustion Engines

James Watt started the steam engine business in collaboration with Matthew Boulton. A number of improvements were made for the application of steam engines including the equipment for converting the reciprocating motion to rotation. However, he prohibited the development of high-pressure steam engines because the high-pressure steam had the potential to cause a dangerous explosion in the high pressure parts such as boilers. However, the use of high pressure was the key technology for downsizing the steam engines. The first steam locomotive utilized a high-pressure steam engine.

The steamboat was invented by Jouffroy d'Abbans in 1783. John Fitch demonstrated the navigation of the steamboat in 1787 although it was commercially unsuccessful. Robert Fulton successfully started the steamboat business operation in 1807. Richard Trevithick developed a high-pressure steam engine for a steam locomotive in 1779. The demonstration of a steam locomotive was carried out to confirm its performance in 1801. However, the locomotive's heavy weight caused accidental damage in the railroad of cast iron. The commercial success of steam locomotive was attributed to George Stephenson, who built the first public railway between Stockton and Darlington in 1825. It should be noted that the commercialization of steamboats and steam locomotives was achieved after incremental improvements that were developed from the basic concept in the original invention.

Reciprocating heat engines have evolved from steam engines to internal combustion engines, and the incremental improvements resulted in the spark ignition engines using the gaseous and volatile fuels. As a result, Étienne Lenoir developed a gas engine in 1860, and Nikolaus Otto developed a four-stroke engine in 1876. An advanced ignition system for compression ignition was developed by Rudolf Diesel in 1893. Further advances in thermal efficiency was achieved by the development of turbine engines because the pressurized gas was capable of rotating multistage turbine rotors while the thermal energy produced in reciprocating engines was converted to mechanical energy with a single stroke of the piston. Heat engines with rotary motion were utilized in steam turbines and gas turbines. The modern steam turbine was invented in 1884 by Charles Parsons after John Barber had received the first patent for primitive turbine engines in 1791. The first steam turbine-powered steamship was built in 1894, and the first successful gas turbine was built by Aegidius Elling in 1903. A variety of heat engines are now available for the power sources of transportation system [7, 8]. Small vehicles require compact engines, and gasoline engines are currently used in numerous passenger cars. Higher efficiency is required for large commercial vehicles, and most diesel engines are used in trucks and vessels. Jet engines have replaced the propeller mechanism driven by gasoline engines in high-speed aircraft because the jet engines generate extensive power to eject the combustion gas backward. Steam turbines and gas turbines are the major power sources for electric power generation due to the low cost generation of electric power.

### 5.1.3. Machining and the Part Production

The development of steel materials along with the processing technology has contributed to the advancements in heat engines. The steam engine requires the combination of pistons and cylinders to operate smoothly and the valve mechanism for controlling the flow of steam. Machining accuracy for making the precise dimensions of cylinders is required for the Watt's steam engine to maintain the air tightness between piston and cylinder. This was realized with the Wilkinson's boring lathe that had been used for the machining of cannons. The production of interchangeable parts is important for the mass production of industrial products. Advances in machining technology have enabled the manufacture of interchangeable parts. Eli Whitney began the production of small guns combining interchangeable parts in 1798. These parts were produced with the screw-cutting lathe developed by Henry Maudslay in 1797.

The advancement in heat engine technologies is associated with the improvement in material technology because the capability of withstanding high pressure is required for the materials and joint parts of high-pressure steam engines such as boilers, pistons, and cylinders. The parts in an internal combustion engine are required to withstand the pressure and temperature of the explosion because intermittent explosive combustion occurs inside the cylinder. In a gas turbine, the development of high temperature alloy and components are particularly important because the hot parts are continuously exposed to high temperatures. The improvement in the thermal efficiency of gas turbines is associated with the technological advances in high temperature materials and the cooling technology of components.

## 5.2. Electric and Communication Technologies

Electrical technology made considerable progress in the 19th century.Extensive scientific knowledge had been accumulated prior to the technological progress [9]. Although the existence of static electricity has been known since ancient times, the scientific knowledge regarding electricity is limited because static electricity discharges in a moment. Investigation on the detailed nature of electricity was started with the direct current generation since the invention of the voltaic pile by Alessandro Volta in 1800. The chemical action of electricity was intensively investigated because the direct current was produced in the voltaic pile as a result of chemical reactions. The relationship between electricity and magnetism was formulated in Maxwell's equations which predicted the electromagnetic wave. Scientific knowledge of electromagnetic induction was theoretically applied to electric power generators and electric motors. The discovery of the electromagnetic wave was applied to wireless communication such as telegram, radio broadcasting and mobile phones.

Developments in electrical technology have enhanced the progress in electric materials and electric parts used for electric applications. These innovations were attributed to Thomas Edison, who developed incandescent light bulbs to start the power generation business. The major historical developments in electric science and technology since the invention of the voltaic pile are summarized in Table 5.2.

In the field of electrical technology, the valuable scientific knowledge, including the nature of electric current and the relationship between electricity and magnetism, was accumulated using the voltaic pile during the preliminary stages of technological development. The discovered phenomena were summarized in theoretical framework. Ingenuity has contributed greatly to the initial progress in electric technologies because the developmental goals in electric technologies are theoretically predictable from the theoretical framework. **This has been formulated in the Maxwell's equations.**

### 5.2.1. Chemical Action of Electricity

Direct electric current promotes chemical reactions because direct electric current is generated by the oxidation of zinc metal in the electrochemical cell invented by Volta. William Nicholson and Anthony Carlisle succeeded in decomposing water into hydrogen and oxygen by electrolysis in 1800, and Luigi Brugnatelli invented electroplating in 1805.

**Table 5.2. Historical developments in electric science and technology**

| Year | Achievements (Contributor) |
|---|---|
| 1800 | Invention of the voltaic pile (Alessandro Volta) |
| 1800 | Electrolysis of water into oxygen and hydrogen gas (William Nicholson and Anthony Carlisle) |
| 1804 | Invention of electroplating (Luigi Brugnatelli) |
| 1807 | Isolation of potassium and sodium by electrolysis (Humphry Davy) |
| 1820 | Discovery of induced magnetic field around the electric current (Hans Christian Oersted) |
| 1825 | Invention of electromagnet (William Sturgeon) |
| 1831 | Discovery of electromagnetic induction (Michel Faraday) |
| 1864 | Suggestion of the existence of electromagnetic waves (James Clerk Maxwell) |
| 1882 | Commercialization of electric lighting (Thomas Edison) |
| 1887 | Verification of electromagnetic wave (Heinrich Hertz) |
| 1901 | Success in the communication test across the Atlantic Ocean (Guglielmo Marconi) |
| 1906 | Radio broadcast (Reginald Fessenden) |

In addition, Humphry Davy discovered the new elements of potassium and sodium in 1807 by the electrolysis of molten sodium carbonate and potassium carbonate. The chemical action of electricity has been applied to manufacturing aluminum, chlor-alkali process and the secondary battery charging.

### 5.2.2. Electricity and Magnetism

The induced magnetic field around the electric current was discovered by Hans Christian Oersted in 1820. The magnetic effect of the electric current is intensified when the iron core is placed inside of coiled wires. This discovery was directly applied to the invention of the electromagnet by William Sturgeon in 1825. In 1831, Michel Faraday discovered the phenomenon of electromagnetic induction during which the current is generated due to the variation in magnetic field. As a result, the development of electric generators began.

Electromagnetic induction in the coil placed near the rotating permanent magnet is the common method of generating electricity. An electric generator works as an electric motor when the electric current is applied to the coil in the generator because the coil works as electromagnet resulting in the rotation of a magnetic rotor. The practical generator was produced by Antonio Pacinotti in 1860, while the commercial success was achieved in 1869 by Zenobe Gramme who produced the generator for lightening arc lamps. Thomas Edison began the electric light business in 1882 using incandescent lamps. An electric power plant driven by a steam engine was built at Pearl Street in New York City to supply direct current. In the 20th century, the application of electricity has spread to a variety of convenient products including electric fans, vacuum cleaners, washing machines and other advanced electric equipment.

Changes in the current flowing through the wire produce a change in the orientation of the compass placed near the wire. This was applied to the communication while requiring a number of wires for sending information, and incremental improvements have been conducted to reduce the number of wires.

The telegraph using Morse code was an innovative technology to send information in the form of on-off signals through a wire. The telegraph has been successfully used due to the simplicity of recording information. In the first operation of telegraph in 1844, indentations corresponding to the on-off signals were made on a paper tape at the receiver when the electrical current was transmitted.

### 5.2.3. Wireless Communication

James Clerk Maxwell summarized the scientific knowledge of electricity and magnetism and suggested the existence of electromagnetic waves in 1864. An electromagnetic wave is the change in an electric field that induces the changes in the surrounding magnetic field, and the magnetic field variations induce the variations in the surrounding electric field.

As a result, the paired fluctuations of the magnetic and electric fields propagate an electromagnetic wave. Accordingly, the short circuit between the high-voltage electrodes generates electromagnetic waves due to the large fluctuation in the electric field occurring at the moment of the short circuit. The presence of electromagnetic waves was verified by Heinrich Hertz in 1887. A telegraph using the electromagnetic wave was developed later. Guglielmo Marconi succeeded in the communication test across the Atlantic Ocean in 1901.

Wireless telegraphy conveys the on-off information using electromagnetic waves. An advanced method has been developed for sending information by modulating the high-frequency electromagnetic waves [10]. Radio broadcasting with amplitude modulation sends the sound wave by changing the intensity of sound superimposed on the high frequency radio waves. The radio receivers extract the audio waves by removing the high-frequency component.

The first radio broadcast was made by Reginald Fessenden in 1906. In 1933, Edwin Armstrong patented the radio broadcast with frequency modulation and as a result, FM radio broadcasting began in 1937. The wireless transmission technology has developed from radio broadcasting to TV broadcasting to send both audio and visual information. Broadcasting technology coupled with the digital information has developed with the advance in computer technology. The digitalized information is transmitted between senders and receivers while the additional processing is required for conversion between analog and digital information.

Radar was another application of radio waves. The first practical radar was produced in 1935. Radar utilized the electromagnetic wave that was used for radio broadcasting. The development of microwave generators such as a magnetron has improved the resolution of radar because the electromagnetic wave of short-wavelength improves the resolution of radar. Percy Spencer discovered the unexpected effect of microwaves to heat moisture. As a result, the microwave oven was first produced in 1947.

## 5.3. Atomic Energy

Research on nuclear technology has been conducted since the discovery of the X-ray. The nature of radiation and radioactive elements has been explored. The discovery of X-ray was directly applied to medical examinations. The potential of nuclear reactors and atomic bombs were facilitated by the phenomenon of nuclear fission of uranium [11]. The development of atomic energy is based on the scientific research independent of the application, and the possible application was theoretically predicted from the advances in nuclear science.

### 5.3.1. Discoveries of X-Ray and Radioactive Substances

There were numerous advances in nuclear technology during the 20th century. The research was initiated with the accidental discovery of the X-ray in 1895 by Wilhelm Conrad Röntgen [12]. The X-ray beam, an invisible ray generated from the discharge tube, is capable of exposing photographic plates and emitting visible light from fluorescent screens. The strong penetration ability of the X-ray was directly applied to the medical examination in order to visualize the internal structure of the human body. In addition, X-ray crystallography was developed by Peter Paul Ewald and Max von Laue in 1912 for examining the crystal structure of materials. The advanced X-ray tube to produce strong X-ray emissions was developed by William Coolidge in 1913.

Intensive research has been conducted to identify the substance that emits radiation since the discovery of the X-ray. Antoine Henri Becquerel discovered the phenomenon in 1896 because photographic plates were affected with the radiation emitted from uranium salts. In addition, Marie Curie extracted a strong radioactive substance from the pitchblende in 1898 which she named radium. Research on the emissions from the radioactive substance revealed that there are three types of radiation, alpha particles, beta particles and gamma rays. The alpha particle is a positively charged particle consisting of a helium nucleus that has jumped out of the nucleus at the alpha decay of radioactive elements. The beta particle is a negatively charged high-speed electron beam that is produced when a neutron in the nucleus changes to the proton. The gamma ray is emitted as high energy photons as a part of the released energy at the time of radioactive decay. An enormous amount of energy released with the decay of radioactive elements is associated with the mass loss during the decay. The relationship between energy and mass loss has been given by Einstein's theory of special relativity.

### 5.3.2. Nuclear Fission and Atomic Energy

In addition to alpha decay and beta decay, radioactive elements can be collapsed by fission. The fission of uranium was discovered when irradiated with neutrons, and the unstable nuclei that are produced by the neutron absorption cause the nuclear fission. The chain reaction of nuclear fission occurs when the released neutrons at the fission are absorbed in other nuclei to cause the induced fission. The chain reaction of nuclear fission was applied to the development of nuclear reactors and atomic bombs. In nuclear reactors, the chain reaction produces the nuclear fission of uranium-235 accompanied with heat generation, as well as the generation of plutonium-239 from uranium-238. The first atomic reactor was used for plutonium production. This plutonium was used for the atomic bomb dropped on Nagasaki. Heat produced in nuclear reactors is used for driving steam turbines to generate electricity. Nuclear reactors have been installed in atomic submarines and atomic aircraft carriers since the 1950s.

**Table 5.3. Progress in nuclear science and technology**

| Year | Achievements (Contributor) |
|---|---|
| 1895 | Discovery of X-ray (Wilhelm Conrad Röntgen) |
| 1896 | Discovery of radioactivity in uranium (Antoine Henri Becquerel) |
| 1898 | Discovery of radioactive polonium and radium (Marie Curie) |
| 1897 | Discovery of alpha and beta radiations (Ernest Rutherford) |
| 1905 | Theory of special relativity (Albert Einstein) |
| 1932 | Discovery of the neutron (James Chadwick) |
| 1939 | Discovery of nuclear fission (Otto Hahn and Lise Meitner) |
| 1942 | The construction of nuclear reactor (Enrico Fermi) |
| 1945 | Development of nuclear bombs (Manhattan Project) |

However, the application to commercial electric power plants requires cost reductions due to huge cost for safety assurance of atomic reactors. Several test plants were built in the 1950s, and commercial nuclear power plants have been intensively built since the 1970s.

Concerns about nuclear power plants are associated with the health and safety problems. Nuclear proliferation along with an increase in the radioactive waste disposal may increase the risk for nuclear terrorism, and the eradication of nuclear accidents may significantly increase the operational costs in nuclear power plants. Table 5.3 summarized the progress in nuclear science and technology. Note that intensive work has been conducted before the discovery of nuclear fission that has suggested the enormous energy generation from nuclear reactions, and the early stage of investigation was not intended for the application of nuclear energy.

## 5.4. Chemical Products

Experimental repetition is effective for scientific discoveries, and the discoveries of scientific facts have directly contributed to the progress in the fields of chemicals, pharmaceuticals and industrial materials. The selection of the most likely research area is naturally based on the theoretical background, and valuable scientific facts are often discovered after numerous attempts. However, the discoveries are not always theoretically intended, and some important facts are accidentally discovered. Unexpected discoveries have greatly promoted the technical progresses in chemical products, and the process has been incrementally improved with numerous trial-and-error repetitions.

### 5.4.1. Explosives

Black powder, a mixture of potassium nitrate, carbon and sulfur, is an explosive that uses the oxidizing power of potassium nitrate for rapid combustion. Black powder was used for the matchlock ignition while the black powder produces smoke at combustion. This is a drawback in using black powder because the shooting location is easily found with the generation of smoke. The generation of smoke is suppressed with guncotton, which is cellulose nitrate produced from cotton by treating cellulose in a mixture of concentrated nitric acid and concentrated sulfuric acid. The smokeless gunpowder has been successfully used in place of black powder.

The main component of explosives is a chemical substance that promotes rapid oxidation reactions by releasing oxygen easily. The candidates are theoretically selected from substances having excess oxygen in their molecular structure, such as potassium nitrate, ammonium nitrate, nitroglycerin, nitrocellulose, trinitrotoluene, picric acid, ammonium perchlorate and acetone peroxide [13]. Nitroglycerin with a great explosive power was discovered by Ascanio Sobrero in 1846 although the nature of nitroglycerin is too sensitive for explosion. The sensitivity reduction is important for developing the explosives practically used because nitroglycerin causes an unexpected explosion initiated by heat and vibration. In 1866, Alfred Nobel successfully invented dynamite, based on the discovery that the sensitivity to the explosion is reduced to the appropriate level by the impregnation in diatomaceous earth, and the ignition was controllable with the detonator.

### 5.4.2. Silver Halide Photography

Light passing through the pinhole produces a reverse image of upside down, and the image transcription produces the realistic drawings on paper. This is the principle of the Camera Obscura that was a tool for drawing a realistic picture in the 15th century. Convex was used in place of the pinhole in 1568, and the image produced with the convex is brighter than the pinhole image. The image can be fixed by tracing the outline of the image projected on the screen of frosted glass through the lens.

Johann Schulze demonstrated in 1725 that silver salts are darkened with the exposure. The image produced with convex is temporarily fixed on the photosensitive material containing silver salts by bright light exposure. However, the image soon disappears because further exposure to light makes the image completely dark. The problems to be solved in the development of silver halide photography are (i) to create the visible image in a short exposure time and (ii) to fix the image without further darkening. Louis Daguerre successfully solved the problems in 1835, based on the prior work developed by Joseph Nicéphore Niépce. The first step is the short time exposure of a photographic plate. This is a copper plate that is coated with silver iodide to produce a positive picture, while no visible image is produced in the short exposure time. The second step is the exposure to mercury vapor, and the visible image is produced on the plate. This is because mercury vapor produces an amalgam of the latent image of silver, and the amalgam promotes the chemical reduction of silver halide to silver metal. The image is fixed with the removal of the residual silver halide. The chemical compound suitable for photographic fixer is a sodium thiosulfate solution, which has been found by John Herschel in 1839 and successfully dissolves the residual silver halide (AgX) in the chemical reaction as follows.

$$2\ Na_2S_2O_3 + AgX \rightarrow Na_3[Ag(S_2O_3)_2] + NaX$$

Louis Daguerre released the daguerreotype technology to produce a positive image in 1839. William Henry Fox Talbot developed a photographic technique to create a negative image around the same time with the positive images reproducible from the negative image on the photographic paper. Photographic technology has since advanced in the quality of photographs and the convenience in taking photographs. The Lumière brothers developed the color photography process in 1907, the instant camera was released in 1972, and solid state image sensors, instead of silver halide photography, were used in the still video camera released in 1981.

## 5.5. Pharmaceutical Products

Important functions of pharmaceutical products are (i) the reduction of pain and suffering from disease and injury, (ii) the prevention of the outbreak of disease, (iii) the medical treatment of disease. Various medicinal herbs have been empirically known to be effective for reducing the symptoms of disease, and the variolation to prevent from smallpox has a long history. However, the further development in pharmaceutical products is associated with advancements in scientific research, including the identification of pathogens that cause disease and affect the working mechanism of cells and organs [5]. Antibiotics are effective for infectious diseases. Pharmaceuticals to adjust the function of the human body are effective for relieving lifestyle diseases. Development of pharmaceutical products was facilitated by trial-and-error approaches including accidental discoveries as well as technological development in extracting the active ingredients from natural substances. The most recent developments are associated with advances in chemical synthesis and life science. A target drug action is identified to design the target drug, and a large number of compounds are synthesized in a short time with the assistance of combinatorial chemistry. Although the development of pharmaceuticals has been considerably promoted with serendipity, the accumulation of scientific knowledge on the biological mechanisms has increased the contribution of the theoretical approach.

### 5.5.1. Drugs for Improving Medical Symptoms

In 1830, the antipyretic effect of willow was revealed to be caused by salicylic acid. In 1852, the salicylic acid was chemically synthesized and was provided for a prescription as anti-inflammatory drugs or antipyretics while stomach pain occurred as a serious side effect due to the highly acidic characteristic of salicylic acid. In 1897, the serious side effect was reduced by the synthesis of acetylsalicylic acid which is the weakened acid, and the anti-inflammatory drug of acetylsalicylic acid has been produced under the trade name of aspirin.

The degradation in biological functions causes symptoms such as diabetes, hypertension and hyperuricemia. Lifestyle diseases, including cancer and heart disease, are associated with the degradation in the biological functions. Although the occurrence of such symptoms depends largely on lifestyle, the administration of appropriate drugs improves the medical symptoms. In fact, insulin lowers the blood glucose level, and allopurinol prevents the production of uric acid. Insulin was extracted from the pancreas in 1921, and the insulin obtained from cows and pigs was administered to patients with diabetes. The development in recombinant DNA techniques enabled the production of synthetic human insulin in 1980, and the side effects due to the animal insulin were reduced.

### 5.5.2. Vaccinations

Patients who have recovered from smallpox never suffer from smallpox again while the lethal infection rate of smallpox is 20 – 40%. Therefore, the infection of smallpox with mild symptoms may reduce the risk of death. The inoculation of the scar tissue taken from the patients who have been cured from smallpox to healthy people was actually conducted in China about 1000 BC [14]. Most of them recover gently with the acquisition of immunity while the initial symptoms of smallpox appear by the variolation. The side-effect is to cause ill patients while the lethal infection rate of variolation is about 1%. Edward Jenner thought that human infectious diseases originated from domestic animals. He verified that the immunity of smallpox was acquired by the inoculation of pus collected from cattle suffering from cowpox in 1796. This was the beginning of the smallpox vaccine using cowpox pus, and the various vaccines have been developed for protecting from other diseases. Note that the technical aspects of developing vaccines are to weaken the toxicity of viruses and bacteria causing infections.

The ability to cause serious diseases is attenuated with cultured pathogens. Louis Pasteur has discovered attenuated cholera pathogens, which are capable of providing immunity without causing diseases, after continuing the cultivation of pathogens in 1880. Pasteur produced the anthrax prevention in 1881 and the live attenuated rabies vaccine in 1885. Albert Calmette and Camille Guérin developed the Bacillus Calmette–Guérin (BCG), which is a vaccine against tuberculosis, and the attenuated bacillus strain was produced through long-term cultivation for 13 years. The basic technology of vaccination was developed by Jenner and Pasteur, and it has been applied to the prevention of various infectious diseases.

### 5.5.3. Antibiotics and Antibacterial Drugs

A vaccine is effective for the prevention of disease, and inoculation produces an antibody to the viruses and bacteria that cause the disease. Direct injection of antibodies to the patient may be effective for the medical treatment of disease, and serum therapy has developed. The antibody is produced in the blood of vaccinated animals, typically horses, and the serum containing the antibody is extracted to be used for the medical treatment of patients. However, the serum extracted from the blood contains impurities that may cause side effects. Further advancement has been made by the production of monoclonal antibody drugs, which are the pure antibody consisting of a single immunoglobulin.

Alexander Fleming discovered penicillin in 1928. The discovery of penicillin was associated with the careful observation of a contaminated Petri dish that the mold had created a bacteria-free circle around itself. Fleming noticed that the substance produced from the blue mold has the capability of killing staphylococcus, and the substance was extracted and named penicillin in 1929. The discovery of penicillin paved the way for medical applications of antibiotics. The technological development to extract and purify the penicillin from the cultured blue mold was conducted in 1945 by Howard Walter Florey. A variety of antibiotics have been explored and many antibiotics including streptomycin have been discovered. Penicillin exhibits toxicity to eubacteria because it inhibits the synthesis of the cell wall. Low toxicity to humans is due to the fact that there are no cell walls in the human body. Penicillin is a typical antibacterial drug. The other typical antibacterial drug is a sulfa drug that is chemically synthesized. An antiviral drug is a drug that inhibits the growth of the influenza virus, HIV virus, and hepatitis virus. Most anti-cancer agents affect the growth of cells by interfering with the replication of DNA. This is the reason why the anti-cancer agent is used for attacking the cancer cells that grow actively though it is harmful for the healthy cells that are actively growing.

## 5.6. Polymeric Materials

Organic substances derived from natural plants and animals have been used for foods, fuels and industrial materials. Timber has been used as a structural material for housing, furniture and mechanical equipment. Natural fiber products have been used for clothing, and ivory and tortoiseshell have been precious handicraft materials. The advance in chemical technologies has enabled the synthesis of organic materials, and the synthesized fibers including regenerated cellulose fibers and chemical fibers are commonly used in clothing. In the development of synthetic fibers similar to silk, the candidate molecules for polymerization were theoretically selected from the molecular groups of polyamide and polyester, whereas the key technology for producing fiber materials was accidentally discovered. High-strength fiber was produced by stretching the viscous materials, and the molecule alignment by stretching was unpredictable at the time. The synthesized resins are used for the substitute of expensive ivory and tortoiseshell.

New classes of polymeric materials have developed. The watertight properties of plastic films are applied to packaging and shopping bags [15, 16]. In addition, advanced materials having unique properties such as Teflon and conductive polymers have been developed. Furthermore, advanced fibers such as carbon fiber and silicon carbide fibers have been developed on the basis of polymer chemistry. Table 5.4 summarizes the major achievements in industrial polymers. Most plastic materials were synthesized in the early and middle 20th century. Their development has been theoretically promoted with the hypothesis proposed by Hermann Staudinger that polymers consisted of long atomic chains held together by covalent bonds. In addition, the discovery of a polymerization catalyst has significantly contributed to the synthesis of advanced polymeric materials while the stretching technology has played an important role in the development of chemical fiber.

**Table 5.4. Major achievements in industrial polymers**

| Year | Achievements (Contributor) |
|---|---|
| 1870 | Application of celluloid to billiard balls (John Hyatt) |
| 1908 | Viscose rayon (Brandon Berger) |
| 1910 | Production of Bakelite (Leo Baekeland) |
| 1910 | Synthesized butadiene rubber (Sergei Lebedev) |
| 1930 | Development of Neoprene (Wallace Carothers) |
| 1938 | Production of Nylon fiber (Wallace Carothers) |
| 1939 | Production of LDPE (Michael Perrin) |
| 1953 | Development of HDPE (Karl Ziegler) |
| 1954 | Development of PP (Giulio Natta) |

### 5.6.1. Natural and Synthetic Resins

A variety of organic materials have been used for handicrafts. The secretion of shellac is a resinous substance used for the varnish coating on violins. Ivory is a composite material consisting of hydroxyapatite and collagen, and the shell of hawksbill tortoise comprises hard proteins called keratin. The coagulated latex obtained from rubber trees was applied to an eraser, and the application was later expanded to raincoats and rubber tires with the advance in chemical modification. Technological progress in synthetic resins has successfully replaced the expensive ivory with celluloid, and further advances result in the production of general-purpose plastics, such as polyethylene, polypropylene, polystyrene and polyvinyl chloride. A wide variety of plastic materials are used in various products, including polyethylene shopping bags, lapping films and plastic containers.

Celluloid is a product of nitrocellulose mixed with camphor as a plasticizer that is obtained from camphor trees. The first application of celluloid was billiard balls that were substituted for ivory in 1870. Bakelite is a thermosetting resin made from phenol and formaldehyde, developed as an alternative to expensive shellac in 1907 with production starting in 1910. Urea formaldehyde resin is the thermosetting resin produced by the polymerization of urea and formaldehyde, invented in 1920. Charles Goodyear patented the vulcanization process to stabilize rubber in 1844. The discovery was associated with the accidental heating of the natural rubber and sulfur mixture. The main component of natural rubber is polyisoprene, and the improvement of properties of natural rubber has been achieved by the development of chemical rubbers. Butadiene rubber was synthesized from butadiene by Sergei Lebedev in 1910, and neoprene was developed by Carothers in 1930. Styrene butadiene rubber (SBR) produced by copolymerizing styrene and butadiene was developed in the 1930s, and silicone rubber was developed in the 1940s.

### 5.6.2. Regenerated Cellulose Fibers and Chemical Fibers

Natural fiber including plant fiber and animal fiber has been used for clothing. Plant fiber including hemp, flax and cotton consists of cellulose fiber while the available part for textile materials is limited due to the mechanical collection of fibrous materials. Pulp is the cellulose fiber collected by immersing the crushed timber in caustic soda for the elimination of lignin and hemicelluloses, and paper is produced by bleaching pulp with added fillers to give it opacity. Long molecules of cellulose fiber are suitable for clothing, and the regenerated cellulose fibers were produced from the cellulose solutions. In the process of manufacturing viscose rayon, cellulose is reacted with caustic soda and carbon disulfide to produce the viscous liquid of sodium cellulose xanthate dissolved in an alkaline aqueous solution. Filamentous cellulose is formed by extruding from the hole of the nozzle into sulfuric acid. Cellophane, developed by Brandon Berger in 1908, is extruded from the slit in the form of film. Cellulose is also dissolved in a copper sulfate solution containing excess ammonia, and cellulose fiber, named cuprammonium rayon or cupra, is obtained by extruding from the nozzle to the solution of acid or alkaline. The modified cellulose esterified with acetic anhydride is dissolved in acetone, and the acetate fiber, consisting of cellulose bonded with acetyl group, is extruded from a nozzle into hot air to vaporize the solvent.

In contrast, animal fibers such as wool and silk are composed of proteins that are polymerized amino acids. The amino acid is a substance having an amino group and a carboxyl group in the molecule, and the polymerization occurs by the formation of chemical bonding between the amino group and the carboxyl group. Polyamide represented by the nylon fiber is a polymer that is synthesized by coupling the amino group with the carboxyl group. Another candidate for chemical fiber is the polyester, which is characterized by an ester bond in molecular structure formed by the polycondensation of dicarboxylic acids and polyalcohols. The representative polyester is polyethylene terephthalate produced by the polycondensation of ethylene glycol and terephthalic acid. Wallace Carothers studied synthetic polymer in DuPont and synthesized polyamide and polyester, which are viscous liquids unlike silk. The manufacturing process of a synthetic polymer fiber like silk was suggested by the accidental performing to pull out the viscous liquid at the tip of a glass rod. Polymer molecules are orientated by stretching to result in an increase in the strength of the yarn, and the synthetic fiber similar to silk was produced. The nylon fiber, a cold stretched polyamide fiber, has been producedby DuPont since 1938.

### 5.6.3. General-Purpose Plastics

Polymers can be synthesized with the polymerization of organic compounds having a double bond in the molecule, and general-purpose plastics such as polyethylene (PE), polypropylene (PP), polystyrene (PS), and polyvinyl chloride (PVC) are produced in large quantities. Catalysts to promote polymerization are, in particular, important for the development of polyethylene and polypropylene, and the additives for modification are of key importance for improving the properties of polystyrene and polyvinyl chloride materials. Figure 5.2 shows the molecular structures of general-purpose plastics.

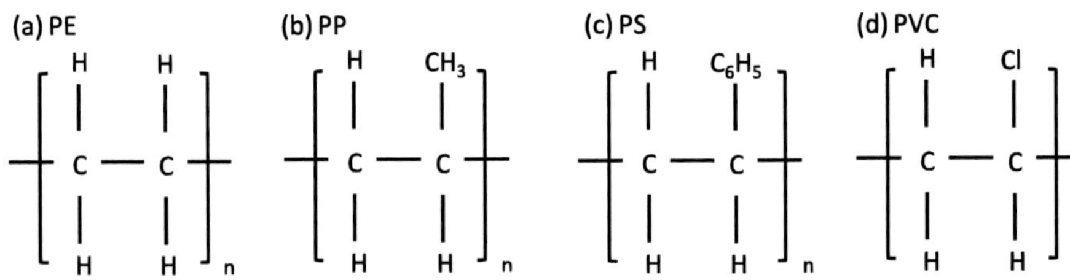


Figure 5.2. Molecular structures of general-purpose plastics, (a) polyethylene, (b) polypropylene, (c) polystyrene, and (d) polyvinyl chloride.

Polyethylene was synthesized in the presence of alkyl lithium compounds at atmospheric pressure by the polymerization of ethylene in 1930, although it was considered a useless byproduct without advancing further research. Thereafter, ICI engineers noticed the generation of polyethylene during the high-pressure experiments of ethylene and also found a leak from the seam of the reactor. This suggests that oxygen works as polymerizing catalyst for polyethylene under high pressures, and the low density polyethylene (LDPE) consisting of branched molecules was developed.

Polyethylene was developed in the UK as insulating coating material for high frequency radar because flexible insulating material covering the cable is important for radar, and the production of LDPE was started in 1939. In the ethylene polymerization process to produce LDPE, oxygen works as a radical initiator in free radical polymerization, and technical improvements in the catalyst currently lead to the use of peroxide, instead of oxygen.

The process of producing high density polyethylene (HDPE), having straight chain with high molecular weight consisting of 10,000 to 100,000 monomers, was developed by Karl Ziegler in 1953. A catalyst consisting of triethylaluminum and titanium tetrachloride is used for manufacturing HDPE under atmospheric pressure, and HDPE was applied to tableware because the high melting point of HDPE is durable for the use in the automatic dishwashing machine. Note that the properties of polymeric materials are governed by the molecular structure and molecular weight, and ultra-high-molecular-weight polyethylene (UHMWPE) has very high strength and impact toughness due to extremely long chains with the molecular weight of several million.

Polypropylene is a thermoplastic resin polymerizing propylene. A methyl group is bound to the alternate carbon chain in polypropylene, and the sequence such as isotactic and syndiotactic regularity produces a high quality crystalline resin. The irregular array of atactic propylene, produced by Ziegler catalyst, is a low-quality amorphous resin. Polypropylene that is generally produced has isotactic regularity with a high stereoregularity. The manufacture was realized by the discovery of the Natta catalyst that is a mixture of dialkyl aluminum chloride ($AlR_2Cl$) and titanium trichloride ($TiCl_3$). Giulio Natta developed the catalyst in 1954, and the commercial production began in 1957.

A polymerization catalyst consisting of titanium chloride and the organic aluminum compound used for the polymerization of HDPE and polypropylene is in general called the Ziegler-Natta catalyst. Figure 5.3 shows the molecular structures of isotactic polypropylene and syndiotactic polypropylene.

Polystyrene is a hard transparent resin obtained by the radical polymerization of styrene that has been produced by BASF since 1930. Polystyrene was discovered from natural resin in 1836. The impact resistance of polystyrene is improved with the addition of synthetic rubber, and the high impact polystyrene (HIPS) contains polybutadiene synthetic rubber. In addition, the acrylonitrile butadiene styrene (ABS) resin is a synthetic resin obtained by copolymerizing styrene and acrylonitrile in the presence of polybutadiene. Another application of polystyrene is the polystyrene foam developed by Ray McIntire, based on the invention by Carl Munters. The Dow Chemical Company started the production of Styrofoam in 1954.

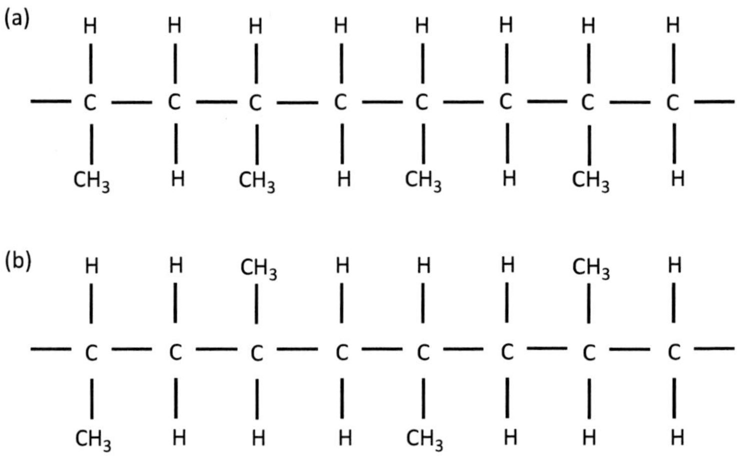

Figure 5.3. Molecular structures of (a) isotactic polypropylene and (b) syndiotactic polypropylene.

Polyvinyl chloride materials normally contain plasticizer and stabilizer because polyvinyl chloride, synthesized from vinyl chloride monomer ($CH_2 = CHCl$), is a hard and fragile material easily degraded by light irradiation. A stabilizer is used for catching the hydrogen chloride generated by photolysis, and plasticizers such as phthalic acid esters are used for softening the material. Therefore, the mechanical properties depend on the addition of plasticizer, and the rigid polyvinyl chloride, containing a small amount of plasticizer, is used for water pipes.

## 5.6.4. Advanced Polymeric Materials

A variety of materials have been developed with the advance in polymer chemistry. Most of them have similar properties to the natural materials while unique properties different from natural products have been found in the advanced polymeric materials such as Teflon and conducting polymers. In addition, the chemical processing of polymer has been applied to the production of carbon fibers and the related materials.

Teflon is a fluorocarbon resin that is the polymer of tetrafluoroethylene, and Teflon is characterized with chemical stability, excellent heat resistance, chemical resistance and a low coefficient of friction. The characteristics have been applied to a variety of products including non-stick pans, the outer clothes of space suits and artificial heart valves. However, the first important application was the manufacture of uranium-235 for the atomic bomb due to the excellent corrosion resistance to uranium hexafluoride. Teflon was discovered by Roy Plunkett at the DuPont research laboratories in 1938 when he opened the valve of a cylinder of tetrafluoroethylene [4]. Since no gas was coming out of the cylinder, he cut the cylinder open to find a white powdery wax. This is Teflon that is polymerized molecules of tetrafluoroethylene. Since Plunkett was aware of the excellent properties of Teflon, the manufacturing process was developed for commercialization in 1946.

Metal exhibits a metallic luster reflecting the visible light due to the presence of free electrons, and the high electric conductivity is applied to the electrode and conductive wires. Electrical conduction in semiconductors results from doping impurities to materials, and the electric carriers are generated responsible for the conduction. Conductive polymer, a kind of semiconductor, has been applied to the electrodes of the capacitor, and the electric conductance is derived from the doped impurities. Since the development of polyacetylene, a variety of conductive polymers have been developed.

Synthesis of polyacetylene powder was reported by Giulio Natta and his coworkers, who polymerized acetylene using a Ziegler-Natta catalyst in 1958. No detailed properties were examined due to the powder form of the synthesized products. Polyacetylene thin film was produced by Hideki Shirakawa in 1967. The successful experiment resulted from an experimental mistake because the concentration of the Ziegler-Natta catalyst was 1000 times thicker than the planned experimental procedure. In 1977, the electrical conductivity comparable to metals was developed in the doped polyacetylene, in which alkali metals are doped as an electron donor and iodine is doped as an electron acceptor.

A number of processes for carbon fibers were investigated during the development of incandescent light bulb filaments, and carbon fibers were produced from cellulose fibers heated in an atmosphere of low oxygen pressure. A composite material of carbon fiber and resin was one of the candidates for high-strength lightweight materials. Intensive research was performed in the late 1950s, focusing on the process from cellulose-based rayon. Polyacrylonitrile was suggested as another candidate to produce the high-performance carbon fiber, and the carbonization process to avoid melting needed to be developed because polyacrylonitrile is thermoplastic. The solution was to form an oxygen bridge between the polymer molecules. This was achieved by low temperature heating in an atmosphere containing oxygen. Using similar technologies, advanced inorganic fibers such as silicon carbide fibers and silicon nitride fibers have been developed.

## 5.7. Electronic Parts and Materials

An electrical circuit is an interconnection of electrical circuit elements such as resistors, capacitors, inductors, transistors, diodes and batteries. The electrical circuit elements are manufactured to exhibit certain characteristics within allowable variations. A further requirement is to miniaturize the dimensions, and the integrated circuit, composed of miniaturized circuit elements such as transistors, diodes, resistors and capacitors, has been developed. On the other hand, various electronic devices including sensors, actuators and displays are used for exerting the necessary function, and the advanced materials having unique properties are of key importance in manufacturing the devices. Semiconductor devices are produced with high-purity materials, and the progress in permanent magnets is due to the discovery of advanced materials [17-19]. In addition, the advance in blue LEDs is associated with the extensive research to improve the manufacturing process, and the discovery of PZT has greatly contributed to the development of piezoelectric devices. Furthermore, the performance of electronic parts such as integrated circuits and multilayer ceramic capacitors has been promoted with the incremental improvements.

### 5.7.1. Semiconductors

High electric conductivity in metals results from free electrons unbound to atoms, and the nature of electric insulators is characterized with electrons strongly bound to the atoms. However, the conductivity of insulators increases at high temperatures due to thermally activated electrons, which are loosely bound to the atoms. The thermal activation intensively occurs in a material having a small band-gap. Therefore, the electrons in semiconductors are activated even at room temperature to allow some degree of electric conductivity.

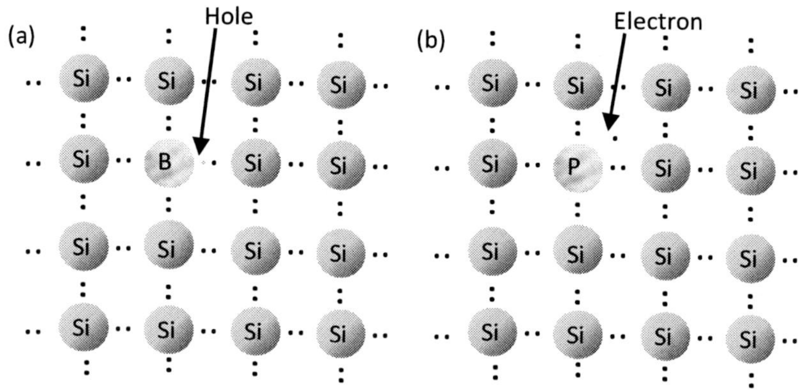


Figure 5.4. Doped semiconductors, (a) p-type semiconductor and (b) n-type semiconductor.

In n-type semiconductors, activated electrons are introduced by doping impurities such as phosphorus and arsenic in silicon. This is because the silicon atom has four valence electrons to form covalent bonds with neighboring silicon atoms while elements such as phosphorus and arsenic have five valence electrons. One excess electron for an impurity atom is loosely bound to allow free movement even at room temperature. In the p-type semiconductor produced with the impurity doping of boron in the silicon, one electron is deficient in the covalent bond for the impurity atom because three valence electrons are supplied by the boron atom. Using the vacant sites produced by impurity doping, an electron bound to silicon easily transfers to the vacant site at room temperature. As a result, the electric conductance in the p-type semiconductors is characterized with the movement of vacant sites, and the vacant sites may be regarded as positive holes because the direction of traveling holes is opposite to that of electrons having a negative charge. Figure 5.4 schematically indicates the doped semiconductors.

## 5.7.2. Diodes and Transistors

A diode has a joined structure of p-type and n-type semiconductors [20]. Electric current is produced when the forward bias voltage is applied to the diode, in which the positive voltage is applied on the p-type semiconductor and the negative voltage is applied on the n-type semiconductor. Under the forward bias, electrons in the n-type semiconductor are trapped in the holes of the p–type semiconductor at the junction. Energy is released as heat and light at the time, and the light emission efficiently occurs in the light-emitting diodes (LEDs). By contrast, the light incident to the diode produces the excited electrons and holes responsible for the electric conduction. This is the principle of photodiodes used for detecting the incident light. Figure 5.5 schematically indicates the structure of the diode, in which the forward bias is applied. Note that the traveling directions of electric charges are opposite when reverse bias is applied, and no current is produced across the p-n junction.

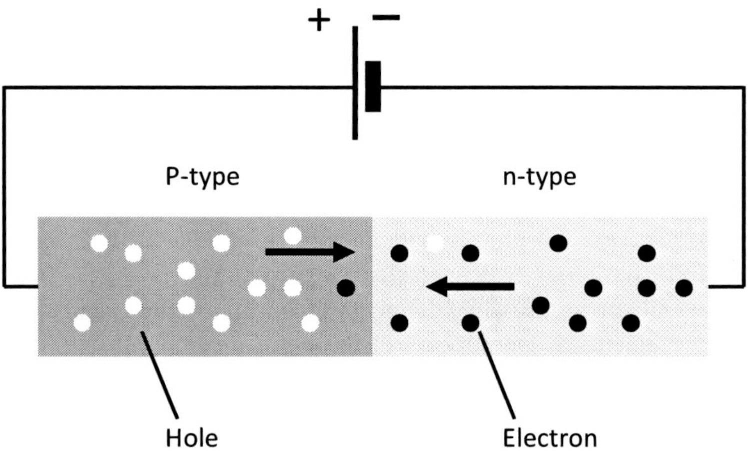


Figure 5.5. Structure of diode indicating that electric current is produced under the forward bias.

**Table 5.5. Band-gaps of some semiconductors**

| Band gap (eV) | | Band gap (eV) | | Band gap (eV) | |
|---|---|---|---|---|---|
| AlN | 6.3 | GaN | 3.44 | Diamond | 5.43 |
| AlP | 2.45 | GaP | 2.26 | Si | 1.11 |
| AlAs | 2.16 | GaAs | 1.43 | Ge | 0.67 |
| AlSb | 1.6 | GaSb | 0.726 | | |

The wavelength of light emitted from the diode is associated with the band gap, and the wavelength of light emission becomes smaller as the band-gap becomes larger. Table 5.5 lists the band-gap of some semiconductors. Gallium nitride is a typical wide band-gap semiconductor, and the blue light is emitted from the GaN LEDs. The infrared emission is produced from the semiconductor having a small band-gap, and the infrared LEDs are commonly produced from gallium arsenide based materials. The infrared LEDs are typically used in the remote control units of commercial products including televisions, air conditioners and lighting equipment, and infrared signals are sent from the remote control unit. The infrared signals are received by the photodiode to reproduce the original information for controlling the electric appliances.

A bipolar transistor of n-p-n junction has the sandwiched structure consisting of the thin layer of p-type semiconductor between two n-type semiconductors. No current is produced when the DC voltage is applied to both ends because the presence of the intermediate thin layer inhibits the electric current.

However, the current is generated when positive voltage is applied to the thin layer of the p-type semiconductor. This is basically the same mechanism as a triode tube invented by Lee De Forest in 1906. The junction transistor was invented by William Shockley, and the integrated circuit contains the miniaturized circuit elements, composed of transistors, resistors and capacitors, formed on the silicon semiconductor. The characteristics of transistors are used for the signal amplification in analog circuits, and the amplification function is used as the switching operation in the digital circuits.

### 5.7.3. Blue Light Emitting Diode and Blue Light Laser

A study with the objective of developing the blue LED was conducted in the 1980s. High luminous efficiency was achieved with a semiconductor crystal having few defects developed on a substrate, and the GaN crystal with few defects was produced with an AlN buffer layer on a sapphire substrate. Further improvement was made by the modification of the electronic structure at the p-n junction through adjusting the chemical composition of the diode and the intermediate layer in the p-n junction. Shuji Nakamura of Nichia Chemical Industries developed blue LEDs having high external quantum efficiency [21]. Nichia Chemical Industries commercialized blue LEDs in 1993. The blue LED has been applied to signals, displays, and lighting. Furthermore, Nakamura developed a blue semiconductor laser which was commercialized in 1999. Blu-ray Disc using a blue semiconductor laser was commercialized in 2002.

Table 5.6 summarizes the major achievements in blue LEDs and blue semiconductor lasers. The progress in blue LEDs has been achieved by the incremental improvements of prior developments, and the blue semiconductor laser is an evolved version of the blue light emitting diode. The progress has been achieved with intensive research, in which numerous ideas are repeatedly tested in trial-and-error approaches.

**Table 5.6. Major achievements in blue LEDs and blue semiconductor lasers**

| Year | Achievements (Contributor) |
|---|---|
| 1989 | The first development of GaN bright blue LED by crystal growth on sapphire substrate with the AlN buffer layer (Isamu Akazaki) |
| 1991 | GaN blue LED with the luminous efficiency of 0.18% using p-n junction (Shuji Nakamura) |
| 1992 | GaN blue LED with the luminous efficiency of 0.22% using double hetero junction (Shuji Nakamura) |
| 1993 | GaN blue LED with the luminous efficiency of 2.7% using the light-emitting layer of GaInN (Shuji Nakamura) |
| 1993 | Commercialization of blue LED (Nichia Chemical Industries) |
| 1995 | GaN blue LED with the efficiency of 9.2% having the light-emitting layer of quantum well structure (Shuji Nakamura) |
| 1996 | Blue semiconductor laser of high-power pulse oscillation (Shuji Nakamura) |
| 1999 | Commercialization of blue semiconductor laser (Nichia Chemical Industries) |
| 2002 | Commercialization of blu-ray Disc using a blue semiconductor laser |

### 5.7.4. Superconductors

Kamerlingh Onnes measured the electrical resistance of mercury at low temperatures and unexpectedly discovered the superconductivity with a resistance of zero below the temperature of 4.2K. Electrical resistance had been expected to decrease with a decrease in the temperature, and the zero resistance was expected to occur at absolute zero temperature. The critical temperature for superconducting transition varies depending on the substances, as shown in Table 5.7.

Before 1986, the materials of high critical temperatures were known in the group of inter-metallic compounds including Nb. Once the superconductivity in the system of La-Ba-Cu-O was discovered, intensive research activities have revealed various oxide compounds containing Cu that exhibit the critical temperatures exceeding liquid nitrogen temperature. In addition, the materials having high critical temperature have been discovered in a new class of materials such as $MgB_2$ and $LaFeAsO_{0.9}F_{0.1}$.

**Table 5.7. Critical temperature of superconductors**

| Critical temperature (K) | |
|---|---|
| Hg | 4.2 |
| Nb | 9.2 |
| NbTi | 10 |
| $LiTi_2O_4$ | 11 |
| $Nb_3Sn$ | 18 |
| $Nb_3Ge$ | 23 |
| $LaFeAsO_{0.9}F_{0.1}$ | 26 |
| $MgB_2$ | 39 |
| $YBa_2Cu_3O_7$ | 93 |
| $Bi_2Sr_2Ca_2Cu_3O_{10}$ | 110 |
| $HgBa_2Ca_2Cu_3O_x$ | 133 |

The first high-temperature superconductor was discovered by Johannes Bednorz and Alexander Muller, who were in the IBM Zurich Research Laboratory investigating the ferroelectric materials to examine the electrical resistance of the La-Ba-Cu-O system at low temperatures. Their experimental result suggested the critical temperature of superconductivity near 30K in their original publication in June 1986.

Since the high-temperature superconductivity was confirmed by a research group in the University of Tokyo in December 1986, the research has been actively conducted worldwide, resulting in the discovery of the high-temperature superconductor of $YBa_2Cu_3O_7$ that has a critical temperature above liquid nitrogen temperature reported in February 1987 [22]. The superconducting cable that comprises the super conducting $Bi_2Sr_2Ca_2Cu_3O_{10}$ wires embedded in a silver pipe is under development, and the cable is cooled by liquid nitrogen to 77K.

## 5.7.5. Magnetic Materials

The nature of magnetite to attract iron has been known since ancient times. The electromagnet was invented in the 19th century. The magnetic force is retained in the electromagnet in some cases even after removing the current. This is because the iron core becomes the permanent magnet, and the magnetic properties have been explored for a variety of ferrous alloys. Based on the pioneering work to develop the strong magnets, the Alnico magnet was developed. In addition, the investigation of oxide magnets, similar to the magnetite, led to the discoveries of barium ferrite ($BaFe_{12}O_{19}$) and strontium ferrite ($SrFe_{12}O_{19}$). Ferrous alloy magnets are characterized by high residual magnetization and low coercivity, and ferrite magnets have high coercive force and low residual magnetization.

Rare earth magnets are characterized with high residual magnetization and high coercive force. The first generation of rare earth magnet was $SmCo_5$ and $Sm_2Co_7$, and the second generation was the neodymium magnet ($Nd_2Fe_{14}B$) discovered by Masato Sagawa in 1983. The discovery of permanent magnet materials with excellent characteristics such as ferrite and rare earth magnets were directly linked to the development of a powerful motor. Neodymium magnet and ferrite magnet are widely used in DC motors and permanent magnet synchronous motors.

Magnetic materials having low coercivity are used for the core of the transformer and the electromagnet. High frequency operation such as magnetic head core increases eddy current loss, and magnetic material with high electrical resistance is preferable for reducing the eddy current loss. High-performance magnetic heads have been produced with Mn-Zn ferrite, and Ni-Zn ferrite having a lower electric resistance was developed for the use in higher frequencies.

## 5.7.6. Dielectric Materials

Materials of high dielectric constant are advantageous in developing small capacitors because the amount of electric charge stored in capacitors is greater in materials of higher dielectric constants, shorter distances between the electrodes, and wider electrode areas. The development of ceramic capacitors has been promoted with the discovery of barium titanate ($BaTiO_3$), and a further advance was made by the incremental improvements in the process technology towards the development of multilayer ceramic capacitors. In the 1940s, barium titanate was revealed to have an abnormally high dielectric constant due to ferroelectricity, and the chemical composition has been modified to reduce the temperature dependence on dielectric constant.

Electric fields applied to the ferroelectric material cause the displacement of constituent atoms to produce polarization, and the displacement produces the dimensional change of crystal. Piezoelectricity is a phenomenon to generate dimensional changes produced by the application of an electric field to the material, and the dimensional change in piezoelectric materials produces the high voltage due to the induced polarization. An excellent piezoelectric material of PZT that has a chemical composition of Pb ($Zr_x$, $Ti_{1-x}$) $O_3$ with x = 0.525, was found in 1952. PZT has been applied to small speakers, piezoelectric igniters for gas appliances, surface acoustic wave filters, ink jet printers, and piezoelectric injectors of the diesel engines. Excellent ferroelectric and piezoelectric materials have been discovered in the end of the intensive research in the most likely research area.

## REFERENCES

[1] Moore, A. D., *Invention, Discovery, and Creativity*, Doubleday, NY, 1969.
[2] Jewkes, J., Sawers, D. and Stillerman, R., *The Sources of Invention*, Norton and Company, NY, 1971.
[3] Hanson, N. R., *Patterns of Discovery: An Inquiry into the Conceptual Foundations of Science*, Cambridge University Press, Cambridge, 1958.
[4] Roberts, R. M., *Serendipity: Accidental Discoveries in Science*, Wiley, NY, 1989.
[5] Meyers, M. A., *Happy Accidents: Serendipity in Modern Medical Breakthroughs*, Arcade Publishing, 2007.
[6] Lienhard, J. H., *How Invention Begins: Echoes of Old Voices in the Rise of New Machines,* Oxford University Press, Oxford, 2006.
[7] Sandfort, J. F., *Heat Engines: Thermodynamics in Theory and Practice*, Anchor Books, NY, 1962.
[8] Okada, A., *Innovative materials for Automotive Industry*, Nova Science, NY, 2010.
[9] Bernal, J. D., *Science in History*, C. A. Watt, London, 1954.
[10] Maclaurin, W. R., *Invention and Innovation in the Radio Industry*, Arno Press, NY, 1949.
[11] Murray, R. L., *Nuclear Energy*, Butterworth-Heinemann, Oxford, 2008.
[12] Lapp, R. E., *Roads to Discovery*, Harper, NY, 1960.
[13] Davis, T. L., *The Chemistry of Powder and Explosives*, Wiley, NY, 1941.
[14] Challoner, J., *1001 Inventions That Changed the World*, Quintessence, London, 2009.
[15] Osswald, T. A. and Menges, G., *Materials Science of Polymers for Engineers*, Carl Hanser Verlag, NY, 1996.

[16] Young, R. J., and Lovell, P. A., *Introduction to Polymers*, CRC Press, NW, 2011.

[17] White, M. A., *Properties of Materials*, Oxford University Press, NY, 1999.

[18] West, A. R., *Basic Solid State Chemistry*, John Wiley, NJ, 1999.

[19] Smart, L. and Moore, E., *Solid State Chemistry: An Introduction*, CRC Press, FL, 2005.

[20] Sze, S. M., and Lee, M. K., *Semiconductor Devices: Physics and Technology*, Wiley, NJ, 2012.

[21] Nakamura, S., Pearton, S. and Fasol, G., *The Blue Laser Diode: The Complete Story*, Springer, Berlin, 2000.

[22] Hazen, R. M., *The Breakthrough: The Race for the Superconductor*, Simon and Schuster, NY, 1988.

*Chapter 6*

# TECHNICAL ISSUES FOR FURTHER ADVANCES

The most immediate needs are associated with the agricultural and industrial products promoting the survival of humans since the basic human needs originated from the requirements for existence in the food chain. Products of higher performance are preferable for achieving higher levels of satisfaction to enjoy a comfortable and convenient lifestyle. Emergent needs that appear after the material wealth are associated with spiritual satisfaction, which is enhanced by the activities to meet the relationship and self-actualization needs. Spiritual satisfaction is achieved with an intimate relationship in the belonging group such as family and the organization of work, and a satisfactory level is promoted with the activities regarding self-actualization driven by the motivated faithful to their own values.

The enhancement of one's own ability is important for being loved and respected by the other group members. In particular, a high evaluation within the organization is given to the achievements contributing to the organizational objectives while the status in a small group has been traditionally promoted with the economic activities to strengthen the relationships with other members of communities, including the gifts of expecting the return and the conspicuous consumption for displaying the economic power [1]. The economic activities promoted by the relatedness needs may still contribute to the economic growth in societies in which the absolute needs are satisfied because the relative needs to satisfy the desire for superiority are insatiable as indicated by Keynes. The enhancement of one's own ability is indispensable for the needs of self-actualization, and technological advances are expected for extending their own physical and intellectual abilities in post-industrial society.

However, anxiety about the future produces an unsatisfied deficiency since the future is uncertain and unpredictable. The spiritual satisfaction is therefore enhanced by the activities related to the reduction of risk that might occur in the future, including their own future and their descendants. Health maintenance and the accumulation of wealth are useful for assuring their own future, and reducing the future risk is helpful for their descendants. The accumulation of wealth, supported by the economic system to preserve private property, is effective for reducing the economic insecurity in the future while the lowest level is supported with the reliable social security system. Health maintenance is supported with a healthy lifestyle, a healthy environment and medical technology. An envisioned risk derived from industrial development includes environmental degradation and the depletion of available resources because the industrial manufacturing activities enhance the chemical conversion of natural resources to worthy products accompaniedby worthless byproducts.

Industrial products may cause health hazards that appear after a long latency period. Serious problems at the low technical levels of industrial production were health hazards caused by air pollution, water pollution and soil contamination. The release of CFCs (chlorofluorocarbons) into the atmosphere has produced the ozone hole to increase the incidence of skin cancer, and the aspiration of asbestos has increased the risk of mesothelioma cancer. The basic approach for risk issues is to prevent the realization of risk while the technical solution is additionally required when the risk is realized. The risk of accidental damage in nuclear power plants is reduced by strict protection against terrorist attacks and the safe design with appropriate operation against natural disasters such as earthquakes and tsunamis. The victims of nuclear war are potentially reduced with the construction of nuclear fallout shelters. The envisioned risk for descendents is reduced with the preventive activities, including the reduction and nonproliferation of weapons for mass destruction peace-keeping operations environmental conservation and the promotion of sustainable lifestyles while the technical resolutions prepared for the worst cases need to be developed in advance.

## 6.1. Reducing Risks and Uncertainties

The envisioned risk that has frequently occurred is statistically estimated from the probability and magnitude of damage, whereas a great loss may be caused by the accidental damages due to the unpredictable serious events that have presumably a low possibility of occurrence and the huge magnitude of damage such as warfare and natural disasters. The uncertain potential risk is therefore adequately assessed in industries to stabilize business activities, and the preparation for the worst cases is important for organizations to survive for a long period [2].

Since capitalism is based on the business model that investors earn the profit from the business income, the risk for investors is to lose the funds in case that the business income is too small resulting from small sales or large expenses. Accordingly, investments in production facilities are recovered with large amounts of production and sales at reasonable prices. Similarly, since consumers benefit from the long-term use of durable goods, the users of industrial products benefit from long-term quality assurance and maintenance service. Accordingly, in the stage where the performance of industrial products reaches satisfactory levels, the major needs are associated with the long-term use of conventional products rather than the replacement by new products of high-performance.

### 6.1.1. Ensuring Reliability and Durability

Industrial products are designed to satisfy the functions required for customers. The customer chooses the particular product based on cost and performance. The performance includes the initial quality and durability, and the total costs include the purchase price and the operating costs. The purchase price as well as the initial quality is easily evaluated, whereas the total operating costs depend on the duration of use that may end with the obsolescence and the durability of products.

Performance variations in products are evaluated with inspection, and most defective products are removed before shipping. Non-destructive testing including visual inspection is usually performed on all the products, and the sampling inspection is carried out for some products. As a result, the initial quality of products is controlled within a small variation in modern industries. Product durability is evaluated in a test condition that simulates the actual condition of use, and the accelerating test condition is usually employed for shortening the testing period. In many cases, the theoretical background is poor for determining the suitable accelerating test condition, and the actual test condition is determined on the basis of the empirical knowledge supported with the accumulation of test data.

### 6.1.2. Ensuring Safety

The use of products is interrupted with product failure, and the failure may damage the surroundings in the worst cases. The failure of vehicles endangers the passengers, and the failure of production facilities, including chemical plants and nuclear plants, may spread harmful substances to cause health hazards. Accordingly, the technological improvement assuring high safety levels has been intensively made in the fields of vehicles and the production facilities.

The product failure is caused by inappropriate operation, the insufficient performance of the product and an overload beyond design basis. The concept of foolproof design is adopted for avoiding inappropriate operations, and the fail safe design reduces the serious damage caused by the insufficient capability and the overload beyond design basis [3]. In addition, the system reliability depends on the method to combine the subsystems. In case of the series combination of subsystems, the reliability of the whole system is poor because the system reliability is achieved by the normal operation of all the subsystems. On the other hand, the system reliability is high in a parallel system, which is a redundant system combining multiple subsystems in parallel, because the single subsystem that is functioning normally can ensure the reliability of the whole system. Most actual systems have been designed to avoid the serious situations based on the series combination with the appropriate incorporation of the redundant parallel system. Incremental progress in safety design reduces the risk of serious accidents while the additional equipment installed for safety assurance may push up the product costs due to the redundant functions.

Expenditures for ensuring safety are considered in association with the expected value calculated from the magnitude of damages and the probability of occurrence, and the high levels of safety are required for the industrial products that may cause serious damage. Those who might cause serious accidents including aircraft pilots, car drivers and gun holders are well trained in civilized countries to reduce the human errors. The periodical inspections of products in use are effective for maintaining the performance as well as reducing the possibility of accidental damages due to the insufficient capabilities. The inspections are regularly performed on facilities and equipment that may cause the serious problems, such as public facilities, firefighting equipment and transportation systems including elevators. Aircrafts are periodically inspected to avoid in-flight accidents, and the propagations of fatigue cracks are, in particular, carefully inspected because the rupture of aircraft may occur when the crack reaches a critical length. The demand for maintenance services of facilities is increasing since technological progress has supplied large quantities of the complicated products. Appropriate maintenance services have been provided for monitoring the operations of large dump trucks working in mines, and electronic security services have been provided for home security.

## 6.2. Resources and Wastes

Industrial production has increased with the expanding range of resources. Steel production has increased with the use of coke in place of charcoal, and precious natural products have been replaced with synthetic materials. In addition, fossil fuels supply huge energy resources, replacing firewood and charcoal. As a result, large amounts of chemical substances and industrial materials are available for producing a variety of final products, and enormous amounts of energy and resources are consumed in chemical conversion processes and the power sources for driving machines including vehicles and the power generation. In addition, mass production reduces manufacturing costs while large production volumes inevitably generate a huge amount of waste. The prosperity of modern society is thus supported by the consumption of mineral resources including fossil fuels, and the great concern is associated with the environmental impact of wastes and the depletion of available resources. The global environment has changed significantly since the birth of the Earth. The activities of photosynthetic organisms have produced significant environmental changes on the surface of the Earth, and recent human activities are influencing the global environment.

### 6.2.1. Formation of Global Environment

The global environment has changed significantly since the Earth has born as a member of the solar system in 4.6 billion years ago [4]. At this time, the temperature of the Earth was kept high with the frequent collisions of meteorites. The temperature was gradually reduced, and metallic iron sunk down to the center of the Earth to create a nucleus of metallic iron, separated from the rock mantle consisting of magnesium silicate containing iron. The Earth surface had been covered with atmospheric water vapor and carbon dioxide while a decrease in the temperature resulted in the condensation of water vapor to produce the primeval seawater, in which hydrochloric acid was dissolved. The acidic seawater dissolved metallic elements contained in the surrounding rocks and carbon dioxide in the atmosphere. Continental crusts that are rich in silicate contents in comparison with the mantle that have been formed by the isolation from the mantle, and the continental crusts continue to move slowly due to the mantle convection. The heavy metallic elements are generally poor in the surface layer of the Earth while the small parts of various metallic resources are extracted from the vein of host rocks where ore minerals have been precipitated from hot water dissolving mineral resources deep under the ground.

The surface temperature of the Earth is determined by geothermal energy and the radiation from the sun. The geothermal energy, originated from the collapse of the radioactive elements such as uranium and thorium deep in the ground, govern the inner temperature of the Earth, whereas the sunlight radiation governs the surface temperature of the Earth. Furthermore, the surface temperature of the Earth is influenced by the atmosphere and the position of the continents.

**Table 6.1. Events influencing the global environment**

| Year | Events |
|---|---|
| 13.7 billion years BP | Big bang or the birth of universe |
| 4.6 billion years BP | Birth of the solar system including the Earth |
| 2.7-1.9 billion years BP | Intensive deposition of banded iron formations |
| 0.5-0.4 billion years BP | Landing of organisms |
| 0.065 billion years BP | Meteorite impact to terminate the Mesozoic era |

* BP: before present.

The surface temperature has been drastically reduced with the events of the dust generation such as meteorite impacts and volcanic eruptions to block the sunlight. The volcanic winter occurred around 70 thousand years ago with the volcanic eruption at Lake Toba in Sumatra, and the great meteorite impact terminated the warm Mesozoic Era 65 million years ago. The sunlight energy supplied onto the Earth is reduced by the polar continents covered with ice because the ice reflects the sunlight to reduce the energy injected onto the Earth. The current existence of ice sheets in Antarctica and Greenland reduces the surface temperature of the Earth, alternating the glacial and interglacial period. Major events influencing the global environment are summarized in Table 6.1.

### 6.2.2. Biological Activities for Environmental Changes

Organisms were generated in the presence of water, and the evolution of the organisms created the cyanobacteria, resulting in the release of oxygen to the surrounding area. Oxygen released from the photosynthetic cyanobacteria oxidized the soluble $Fe^{2+}$ ions present in sea water to produce the precipitates of iron oxides such as magnetite ($Fe_3O_4$) and hematite ($Fe_2O_3$). This resulted in the deposition of banded iron formations or sedimentary rocks containing iron oxide layers that occurred from 2.7 to 1.9 billion years ago. The oxygen that leaked from seawater has changed the chemical composition of the atmosphere to produce the thin ozone layer in the upper surface of atmosphere. The ozone layer shields ultraviolet rays from the sun to the ground surface. As a result, organisms safely transitioned onto land around 0.5 billion years ago.

The organisms have produced several important resources. Limestone that is mainly used for steel manufacturing and cement production consists of calcium carbonate that is generated from the corpses of ancient organisms, including calcareous plankton, shellfish and corals. Crude oil and coal are generally thought to be from the corpses of ancient microorganisms and plants.

Crude oil is separated to produce a variety of petroleum products including liquefied petroleum gas (LPG), naphtha (or crude gasoline), kerosene, diesel fuel, fuel oil and asphalt. LPG, which is mainly composed of propane and butane, is liquefied by applying pressure and is used for household energy such as heating and cooking. Gasoline for automobiles is modified to increase the octane number, and the crude gasoline is blended with the synthesized fuels of reformed molecules having branches, phenyl rings, and double bonds. Some parts of naphtha are thermally decomposed to small molecules such as ethylene, propylene and butadiene. Kerosene is used for heating and jet fuels. Diesel fuel is utilized for diesel engines in trucks and buses, and fuel oil is used for industrial boilers and fuels for the diesel engines of vessels. Natural gas, mainly composed of methane, is used for thermal power generation and city gas.

Coal is classified based on the amounts and types of carbon. Peat, produced at the earliest stage in the formation of coal, is a soft organic material consisting of partly decayed plant matter together with deposited minerals. Lignite coal is the lowest rank of coal having a fixed-carbon content ranging from 25 to 35 percent, and sub-bituminous coal has a higher fixed-carbon content ranging from 35 to 45 percent. Bituminous coal is a soft coal having a fixed-carbon content ranging from 45 to 86 percent, and anthracite coal is a hard black coal containing the highest fixed-carbon content of 86 to 98 percent. Coal is mainly used as fuel for boilers to generate steam in thermal power generation. The coke made from dry distillation of bituminous coal is used for blast furnaces to produce pig iron by reducing iron ores.

### 6.2.3. Human Activities and the Environmental Issues

The development of industrial technology has consumed vast amounts of resources, which range from the biological products available on the surface of the Earth to the mineral resources deep inside the ground. The environment influences of human activities have increased with the economic development.

Desertification may be the first environmental impact due to human activities by cutting down the forest to use the wooden resources as fuels and construction materials. The use of coal as a substitute for firewood and charcoal was a solution for the shortage of wood resources, and the use of mineral resources including coal has promoted industrial production leading to a society of material wealth. However, the emission of sulfur dioxide gas, generated from the combustion of coal and the roasting of ores, has caused severe air pollution. In addition, the waste and wastewater from mines and manufacturing facilities have contaminated soil and rivers. In the metal refining processes such as copper production, sulfur dioxide is released into the atmosphere by roasting, and the mine pollution degrades the water quality. In the Industrial Revolution, large amounts of sulfur dioxide were emitted into the air from the combustion of coal for heating. The London smog crisis of 1952 was caused by the burning of coal for heating residents, causing the death of more than 4,000 people. The emissions from the copper smelting plant in Swansea, was a serious problem in the 19th century, and the air pollution due to the emission of $SO_X$ and $NO_X$ caused the Yokkaichi asthma in Japan. In addition, air pollution due to $NO_X$ emissions is the cause of photochemical smog under strong sunshine. Cadmium pollution from the copper smelting plants in Japan causes Itai-itai disease because the cadmium was concentrated in the field crops cultivated downstream. In addition, the cause of Minamata disease is the biologically concentrated methyl mercury in fish and shellfish from industrial wastewater released into the sea [5]. The release of CFCs has increased the risk of developing skin cancer by destroying the ozone layer. The major human activities associated with environmental issues are listed in Table 6.2.

**Table 6.2. Human activities associated with the health and environmental issues**

| Year | Health and environmental impact |
|---|---|
| Several thousand years BP | Desertification by cutting down the forest |
| The 19th century | Emission of sulfur dioxide gas from the combustion of coal and the calcinations of ores |
| | Emission of HCl and $H_2S$ gas from the Leblanc process |
| The 20th century | Pollution diseases such as Itai-itai disease, Minamata disease and Yokkaichi asthma |

Harmful emissions have been significantly reduced as a result of the technological progress in wastewater purification and the detoxification of exhaust gas since the effects of environmental pollution have been recognized. The emissions of $SO_X$ and $NO_X$ from manufacturing facilities in developed countries have been significantly reduced with the detoxification processes using lime and ammonia, and the emissions from automobiles have been reduced with the technical advances in fuels and automotive engines. Heavy metals in waste water are processed with neutralizing precipitation, and the organic matter is absorbed in microorganisms to be purified. In addition, there is international collaboration regarding the temperature increase in the atmosphere due to the large amount of carbon dioxide emissions resulting from the consumption of fossil fuels. Another concern is the depletion of underground resources responsible for the high-quality mines because the underground mines producing high-quality resources take precedence over low-quality ones. The consumption of high-quality mines results in an increase in resource prices if it is not accompanied by technological progress, and economic activity may decline.

## REFERENCES

[1] Veblen, T., *The Theory of the Leisure Class*, Macmillan, NY, 1899.

[2] Giarini, O. and Stahel, W.R., *The Limits to Certainty*, Kluwer Academic Press, MA, 1993.

[3] Hitomi, K., *Manufacturing Systems Engineering*, Tayler and Francis, London, 1979.

[4] Brown, C. S., *Big History: From the Big Bang to the Present*, New Press, NY, 2007.

[5] Merson, M. H., Black, R. E. and Mills. A. J., *International Public Health: Diseases, Programs, Systems and Policies*, Jones and Bartlett Learning, MA, 2005.

# INDEX

## D



## E

**F**

## N



## O



## P

**Q**



**R**



**S**

## T

## U



## V



## W



## Y



## Z